PRACTICAL ETHICS FOR NURSES AND NURSING STUDENTS

A Short Reference Manual

Kathryn Schroeter, RN, MS, MA
Clinical Faculty - Bioethics
Medical College of Wisconsin
Surgical Services Education Coordinator
Froedtert Hospital

Arthur Derse, JD, MD
Associate Clinical Professor of Bioethics and Emergency Medicine
Medical College of Wisconsin

Charles Junkerman, MD
Professor Emeritus of Medicine and Bioethics
Medical College of Wisconsin

David Schiedermayer, MD
Professor of Medicine and Bioethics
Medical College of Wisconsin

For my husband, Rodney,
a most practical ethicist
K.S.

University Publishing Group, Inc.
Hagerstown, Maryland 21740
1-800-654-8188
www.upgbooks.com

CONTENTS

INTRODUCTION

The concepts described here are as important to patient care as any diagnostic or management techniques. Evaluative strategies and therapeutic interventions will change frequently, but if the nurse or nursing student can master the art of communication with patients and can learn to identify and resolve ethical problems, she or he will have acquired enduring, career-enhancing skills.

This text contains a brief overview of the information needed for nurses of all types to provide comprehensive, ethical, patient-centered care. Some specialized areas of nursing have been listed because of the ethical issues inherent in these specialties. Also included is a section on legal cases illustrating how ethical issues have been treated in the American justice system. Each section contains concise information on the topic listed. Many of the sections include additional material and a list of a few important references for those who wish to pursue a given subject.

ACKNOWLEDGMENTS

The first author is especially appreciative of the encouragement offered by the editor, Leslie LeBlanc, and of her support for a short, nurse-friendly ethics manual. The expertise and cogent comments of Gloria Taylor, RN, MA, CPTC, UNOS Staff Ethicist; Lisa Thomka, RN, MSN, CNS; and Beth Whitstone, RN, MA, CCRC, have enhanced the accuracy of particular sections and are greatly appreciated. Thorough review by Susan Klapper, MSN, RN, ANP; Colleen A. Malone, RN, BSN; Roberta Pipping, RN, BSN; and Debbie Runyan, RN, BSN, MS, was invaluable and has resulted in a more readable text. The support of the first author's parents; her mentor Dr. Paul R. Hohenfeldt (who motivated her throughout nursing school); as well as the encouragement of other colleagues, Beverly Beine, RN, MS; Marty Fordham, RN, BSN; Gail Kufahl; Jeanne Kunkel, RN, BSN; Ellen K. Murphy, MS, JD, FAAN; Beth L. Rodgers, PhD, RN, FAAN; and Lucy Turkow, RN, BSN, MSM; is also gratefully acknowledged.

The *Code of Ethics for Nurses with Interpretive Statements,* 2001, is used with the kind permission of the ANA.

I. PROFESSIONAL RESPONSIBILITIES

THE NURSE'S ETHICAL DUTIES

The code of ethics for nurses is found in the American Nursing Association (ANA) *Code of Ethics for Nurses with Interpretive Statements,* (2001), which states:

1. The nurse, in all professional relationships, practices with compassion and respect for the inherent dignity, worth and uniqueness of every individual, unrestricted by considerations of social or economic status, personal attributes, or the nature of health problems.
2. The nurse's primary commitment is to the patient, whether an individual, family, group or community.
3. The nurse promotes, advocates for and strives to protect the health, safety and rights of the patient.
4. The nurse is responsible and accountable for individual nursing practice and determines the appropriate delegation of tasks consistent with the nurse's obligation to provide optimum patient care.
5. The nurse owes the same duties to self as to others, including the responsibility to preserve integrity and safety, to maintain competence and to continue personal and professional growth.
6. The nurse participates in establishing, maintaining and improving healthcare environments and conditions of employment conducive to the provision of quality healthcare and consistent with the values of the profession through individual and collective action.
7. The nurse participates in the advancement of the profession through contributions to practice, education, administration, and knowledge development.
8. The nurse collaborates with other health professionals and the public in promoting community, national and international efforts to meet health needs.
9. The profession of nursing, as represented by associations and their members, is responsible for articulating nursing values, for maintaining the integrity of the profession and its practice and for shaping social policy.

Code of Ethics for Nurses with Interpretive Statements, 2001, American Nurses Association, ©2001; used with the kind permission of the ANA. Source: <http://www.ana.org/ethics/#3>.

NURSES' RIGHTS

1. **When caring for patients, nurses have rights that must be respected.**

   - Nurses may refuse to care for a patient when it requires them to perform a treatment or operate equipment that is beyond their training or expertise; it may place a patient in jeopardy.
   - Nurses have the right not to be abused in the workplace.
   - Nurses should not perform tasks that are outside the scope of their practice.
   - Nurses should not perform duties outside state practice acts, even if they are competent to do so.

2. **Nurses may reject an assignment.**

   Nurses should reject assignments that put them or their patients in serious, immediate jeopardy. Nurses' professional obligations to safeguard patients are grounded in the ethical norms of the profession, the *Standards of Clinical Nursing Practice*, and state nurse practice acts.

   When a nurse does not feel personally competent or adequately prepared to carry out a specific function, he or she should do the following:

   - Clarify the assignment.
   - Assess his or her personal capabilities.
   - Identify other options for filling the assignment.
   - Determine the cause of the immediate, serious danger.

   Nurses may be held responsible for the judgments and actions made in the course of their practice.

NURSES' DUTIES

1. Be aware of limitations to scope of practice.
2. Recognize personal accountability.
3. Never jeopardize the standard of care.

WHAT NURSES SHOULD KNOW

1. Patient rights
2. The nurse's obligations as a healthcare provider

3. Hospital policies and procedures
4. Standards of care and practice
5. Community norms

PATIENTS AS INDIVIDUALS

Evaluate individual patients in the following areas:
1. Their comprehension and self-understanding
2. Their values, beliefs, fears, and hopes
3. The seriousness of the condition as reflected in their eyes
4. The need for urgent action
5. How patients' options will affect them physically, psychologically, and socially
6. Patients' ability to participate in their own care

PATIENTS' RIGHTS

Many healthcare organizations have policies on patients' rights. Such policies are likely to include the following items:
1. Patients cannot be denied appropriate care based on their race, religion, cultural background, gender, sexual orientation, marital status, age, newborn status, disability, or source of payment.
2. Patients shall be treated with respect, and their individuality and personal needs shall be respected, including:
   - Privacy
   - Effective pain management
   - Psychosocial needs
   - Spiritual needs
   - Culturally specific needs
3. Patients shall have the opportunity to make healthcare and ethical decisions, in collaboration with healthcare providers.
4. Patients are entitled to know who has the overall responsibility for their care.
5. Patients, or the persons authorized by law, shall receive, from the appropriate healthcare provider, information about their illness, course of treatment, and prognosis for recovery, in terms

they can understand.

6. Patients' medical records, including all computerized medical information, shall be kept confidential as required by state and federal law.

7. Patients, or the persons authorized by law, shall have access to their medical record.

8. Except in emergencies, consent shall be obtained from patients or their legally authorized representatives before they participate in research, or before any diagnostic or surgical procedures are performed.

9. Patients may refuse treatment as permitted by law and shall be informed of the medical consequences of their refusal.

10. Except in emergencies, patients may not be transferred to another facility until:
   - They are given a full explanation for the transfer.
   - Adequate provision is made for their continued care.
   - They are accepted by the receiving institution.

THE FUNDAMENTAL GOALS OF HEALTHCARE

The general goals of medicine and healthcare include:

1. Prevention of disease and untimely death
2. Cure of disease, when possible
3. Improvement or maintenance of functional status when cure is not possible
4. Palliation (relief of pain and suffering), pursuit of a peaceful death, and comfort care in all situations
5. Patient education and counseling

MORAL DECISION MAKING

Nurses must have a realistic understanding of the goals of treatment before they can make good nursing decisions. It is best for the healthcare team and the patient, together, to determine which goals are actually achievable, when possible.

Nurses are responsible for nursing decisions that are not only clinically and technically sound, but also morally appropriate and suitable for the specific problems of the particular patient being treated. The medical (technical) aspects of the decision answer the question, "What *can* be done for this patient?" The moral component involves the patient's wishes and answers the question, "What *ought* to be done for this patient?"

REFERENCES

American Nurses Association. *Code of Ethics for Nurses with Interpretive Statements.* Kansas City, Mo: ANA; 2001.

American Nurses Association. *Standards of Clinical Nursing Practice.* 2nd ed. Kansas City, Mo: ANA; 1998.

Blood-borne diseases—nurses' risks, rights, and responsibilities . . . adapted from the American Nurses Association Workplace Information. *Maine Nurse.* 2000;2(2):16.

Copeland P. Legal forum. Rights and wrongs . . . does a nurse have a duty to treat HIV-infected patients? *Minority Nurse.* 1998; Summer-Fall:34-35.

Daley K. Protecting the public while safeguarding the rights of nurses. *Mass Nurse.* 1999;69(9):3,13.

Elective abortion: court upholds nurse's right to refuse to participate. *Legal Eagle Eye Newsletter for the Nursing Profession.* 1998;6(11):3.

Ellis J. Nurse to nurse. The client's right to know versus the nurse's right to be protected from harm . . . staff identification. *Nursing BC [British Columbia].* 1997;29(5):11-12.

Higginbotham E. Advice of counsel. To refuse triage duty, show potential for patient harm. *RN.* 2001; 64: 74.

Jones W. Nurses' rights equal quality care. *Kentucky Nurse.* 1998;46(4):11. Originally printed in *Am J Nurs.* May 1998;98(5):88.

Kany K. Workplace rights: the wild blue yonder should nurses be floating to unfamiliar units? *Nevada Rnformation.* 2000;9(4):1,23.

Legal issues. HIV litigation update. *AAOHN J.* 1998;46:358-359.

McCullough LB. John Gregory (1724-1773) and the invention of professional relationships in medicine. *J Clin Ethics.* 1997;8(1):11-21.

Professional practice issues . . . floating to an unfamiliar area. *Chart.* 1997;94(4):5.

Quill TE, Cassel CK. Non-abandonment: a central obligation for physicians. *Ann Intern Med.* 1995;122:368-374.

Salladay SA. Ethical problems. Harassment: sex in the CCU. *Nursing.* 2000;30(11):26.

Specifying the goals of medicine. *Hastings Cent Rep.* Nov-Dec1996;26(special supp):9-16.

Steckler SL. Nursing case law update. The Cooper Health System . . . no-solicitation policies. *J Nurs Law.* 2000;7(1):55-64.

Sullivan GH. Advice of counsel. Rights versus consequences of refusing duty. *RN.* 2000;63(12):74.

II. DO NOT RESUSCITATE (DNR)

INFORMATION FOR NURSES

It is important that the issue of cardiopulmonary resuscitation (CPR) be addressed early in the treatment course of a patient with serious illness in whom cardiac or pulmonary arrest is likely. In many cases, the patient will make his or her wishes known to the nurse. The nurse must see that the topic is discussed sensitively with patients, significant others, and the rest of the healthcare providers on the team. It should be emphasized to the patient and/or significant other(s) that comfort and therapeutic measures will remain in effect even though a DNR order is in place.

The rationale and specific provisions for a DNR order should be discussed fully with the nursing staff and with all of the patient's other caregivers so that there are no uncertainties about care plans. Healthcare institutions should have a system in place so that this very important information is not miscommunicated in any way between the healthcare providers, patients, and significant others. Patients are either DNR as clearly specified in the orders or they are full code. "Slow codes," "code grays," "show codes," or "Hollywood codes" are deceptive and place an unfair responsibility on the nursing service. Nurses need to know how to respond in a code situation so that there is no last-minute guesswork in providing appropriate care.

Nursing staff must be familiar with the DNR policies and procedures of their practice settings. This is especially true when DNR orders are to be suspended intraoperatively. Perioperative nurses, as well as perianesthesia nurses, need to know what discussion has taken place with the patient prior to the surgical intervention so that an appropriate response can be initiated should the need for resuscitation arise in the surgical environment. It is also imperative to note when the DNR order goes back into effect if it is suspended intraoperatively.

ATTENTION TO TLC

Many patients and their families fear abandonment when a DNR order is written, so it is important for nurses and nursing students to be attentive and aware of comfort measures. The patient and family must know from the outset that "no code" does not mean "no care."

AUTHORITY FOR DNR

Authority for the decision (in order of importance):

1. Request of a decisional patient (a patient who has decision-making capacity; see section V, p. 25)
2. Dictates of an advance directive
3. Judgment of guardian or healthcare agent appointed in an advance directive

In some states, surrogate laws establish a hierarchy of authority; in others, there is moral authority but no legal authority for the following (if 1 to 3 above are not available):

1. Approval by first-order relatives (spouse, adult children, or parents—in that order)
2. Opinions of other relatives or friends who are able to provide a "substituted judgment" (see section V, p. 25) or who agree upon the best interest of the patient
3. If no relatives or friends are available for consultation, base the decision on medical indications, taking into account whether CPR would further the reasonable personal medical goals of this particular patient.
4. A few states require consent for DNR orders from the decisional patient or from the authorized legal representative (such as a guardian or healthcare agent).

WHAT THE DNR ORDER SHOULD INCLUDE

1. The order should be written by the attending physician or by a house officer at the request of the attending physician.
2. The progress notes should include documentation of:
    - The medical indication for DNR or contraindication to CPR
    - Advice of consultants (if any)
    - Authority for the decision (see above discussion).
3. The order should include specific orders about what treatments are to continue. Specific orders should be in writing to avoid misunderstandings. Ordinarily, DNR simply means "no CPR." DNR orders may have no other significance and may be compatible with

all other modalities of treatment including care in the intensive care unit. On the other hand, a DNR order may be the first step in the withdrawal of other treatment, in which case further clarification is necessary.

DNR ORDERS ON THE BASIS OF FUTILITY

In many institutions, a DNR order may be written by the attending physician on the basis of medical futility (see section XIV, p. 57). Another staff physician should concur in writing, and the justification for this judgment must be clearly indicated in the progress notes. Many policies stipulate that the patient or surrogate need not agree but must be notified. If the patient or surrogate disagrees with the decision, consultation with the institutional ethics committee is appropriate and hospital administration should be notified. A few states require consent for DNR orders from the decisional patient or from the authorized legal representative (such as a guardian or healthcare agent).

ETHICS CONSULTATION

In the event that the authority for DNR is in question or a DNR order written on the basis of futility has created objections on the part of patient, family, or agent, an ethics consultation should be sought for clarification or mediation (see section XXIV, p. 93). Nurses need to be familiar with their facility's system for dealing with ethics issues and with the means by which to activate the assistance when needed.

FURTHER READING

CPR was developed in the 1960s for treatment of sudden cardiac arrest in previously well individuals. Despite warnings that this technique could be inappropriate in other clinical situations, CPR became a default procedure. It was presumed that a patient wanted CPR unless there was a specific request to avoid it. This is a unique presumption in medicine.

Effectiveness of CPR

Public expectations of the success of CPR are quite unrealistic and do not match the statistics. About 15% of hospitalized patients in whom resuscitation is attempted survive to discharge. Furthermore, numerous studies have shown virtually no survival to hospital discharge for patients with overwhelming pneumonia, renal failure, acute stroke, or multiple organ failure who have an in-hospital arrest. Patients older than 70 years of age who have sepsis or metastatic carcinoma or whose resuscitation effort lasts more than 15 minutes are unlikely to survive. Recent research suggests, however, that CPR success varies from one institution to another and that the pre-arrest condition of the patient may be the most important predictor of success.

The best CPR results occur in persons who have a witnessed arrest on the basis of a ventricular dysrhythmia (not asystole) and who are successfully resuscitated within 5 minutes. CPR is successful in 25% of cardiac arrests that result from drug reaction or overdose. Extended CPR (more than 15 minutes) is reasonable in cases of subarachnoid hemorrhage, hypothermia, electric shock, and drug overdose.

Risks (Burdens) of CPR

Of the patients who are successfully resuscitated, 25% to 50% have fractured ribs, fractured sternum, aspiration pneumonia, mediastinal hemorrhage, or pulmonary edema. Up to 10% of those whose CPR is successful may end up in a persistent vegetative state (PVS).

Discussing Patient Wishes Regarding CPR

Patients may bring up the issue of CPR with nurses. It is especially important to address the issue with patients admitted for serious illnesses in which an arrest would not be unlikely and with patients with chronic illnesses whose condition may deteriorate. The wishes of these patients cannot be presumed and, therefore, should be elicited.

Questions about the patient's desire for CPR should be asked in the specific context of that patient's problems. One should avoid questions such as "Do you want us to do everything?" when "everything" is practically impossible for the patient or physician to define. Likewise, the question "Do you want us to start your heart if it stops?" implies falsely that such a result may be certain.

The issue should be approached sensitively and as a part of the overall therapeutic program. The patient may need more information in order to make a decision. The nurse must obtain a physician to provide this information. As with issues of consent, the physician will advise the patient on all aspects of CPR, such as any burdens and risks associated with resuscitation.

If CPR would likely be futile (see section XIV, p. 57), a request for a DNR order should probably follow a discussion emphasizing the positive measures that will be taken for the patient, the reassurance that the patient will not be abandoned, and the promise that all possible comfort measures will be provided.

Some ethicists advocate, with good reason, that DNR should be DNAR (do not attempt resuscitation) because DNR implies that a reasonable degree of success is possible. In patients for whom a DNR or no-CPR order is appropriate, the likelihood of success is usually minimal. To imply otherwise is to mislead the patient and thereby impair his or her autonomous judgment.

If some unforeseen event takes place in the hospital that makes cardiac or pulmonary arrest likely, the subject of code status should be brought up while the patient still has decision-making capacity (if possible). It is not ethical to wait purposefully until an acutely ill patient is no longer decisional in order to discuss code status with a surrogate.

Conflict between the Patient's Desire for "Full Code" and Futility

The American Medical Association (AMA) Council on Judicial and Ethical Affairs has commented that resuscitative efforts "would be considered futile if they could not be expected to achieve the goals expressed by the informed patient. This definition of futility not only respects the autonomy and value judgments of individual patients but also allows for the professional judgment and guidance of physicians who render care to patients" (*JAMA*. 1991; 265: 1868-1871).

Occasionally patients in whom CPR is almost certain to fail insist on the attempt. If the request is clearly irrational (for example, a patient wishes CPR not in an attempt to survive until the arrival of a loved one but simply as part of wanting "everything" done), the physician is under no obligation to provide futile treatment. This right is recognized in law and ethics. Strategies for avoiding this conflict between the patient's desire for futile treatment and the physician's reluctance to use a treatment that is not medically indicated include the following:

1. Avoid using the term "futility," which is hard to define and even more difficult for patients to understand.
2. Determine the patient's goals in the present circumstances.
3. Determine in discussion with the patient or surrogate whether an attempt at resuscitation in light of its benefits and burdens will further these goals.

Relationship of DNR Orders to Advance Directives (ADs)

DNR orders should not be confused with advance directives. ADs require interpretation and need to be incorporated into a treatment plan that includes specific orders consistent with the patient's wishes. This plan may or may not include a DNR order, but DNR is not usually a part of the AD. The existence of a living will does not necessarily indicate that a patient is intent on forgoing CPR.

DNR and the Operating Room (OR)

Anesthesiologists have expressed their discomfort with DNR orders in the OR because an arrest might occur during a procedure in the OR that is not related to the underlying disease, and this arrest may be easily managed with drugs. In this situation, anesthesiologists are reluctant to stand by and watch the patient die. Therefore, DNR policies should be modified so that ordinarily the DNR order is suspended when the patient goes to the OR (or a procedure such as cardiac catheterization) and is reinstituted automatically on discharge from the postanesthesia care unit. The patient should be notified of the policy for placing the DNR order on hold and should have the option of overriding the policy, keeping the DNR order in effect through the procedure.

REFERENCES

American Medical Association, Council on Ethical and Judicial Affairs. Guidelines for appropriate use of do-not-resuscitate orders. *JAMA*. 1991;265:1868-1871.

Hakim RB, et al. Factors associated with do-not-resuscitate orders: patients' preferences, prognoses, and physicians' judgments. *Ann Intern Med*. 1996;125:284-293.

Jayes RL, et al. Do-not-resuscitate orders in intensive care units. *JAMA*. 1993;270:2213-2217.

Kane RS, Burns EA. Cardiopulmonary resuscitation policies in long term care facilities. *J Am Geriatric Soc*. 1997;45:154-157.

Lo B. Unanswered questions about DNR orders. *JAMA*. 1991;265:1874-1875.

Reeder JM. Do-not-resuscitate orders in the operating room. *AORN J*. 1993;57:947-951.

Tomlinson T, Brody H. Futility and the ethics of resuscitation. *JAMA*. 1990;264:1276-1280.

Wenger NS, et al. Patients with DNR orders in the operating room: surgery, resuscitation, and outcomes. *J Clin Ethics*. 1997;8:250-257.

III. WITHDRAWAL OF TREATMENT

WHAT NURSES SHOULD KNOW

Nurses must be able to recognize the difference between *withdrawing* and *withholding* treatment.

1. **Psychological Difference**

   Psychologically, it is easier not to start a treatment than it is to stop it. But a moment's reflection demonstrates that this is illogical—the decision to omit treatment is just as much a willful judgment as the decision to withdraw it.

2. **"Up-Front Barrier"**

   By deciding not to start a specific treatment, clinicians may be erecting an "up-front barrier"—that is, clinicians may be denying in advance a treatment that might possibly be effective. Thus, a decision not to initiate treatment (to withhold treatment) must actually have stronger substantiating reasons than a decision to discontinue (withdraw) treatment that has clearly failed.

3. **Time-Limited Trial**

   When there is some uncertainty as to the effectiveness of a treatment in furthering the patient's goals, the bias clearly must be in favor of a time-limited trial of treatment. If it later turns out to be ineffective and not beneficial for a particular patient in a given circumstance, the treatment can be stopped. Use of this model gives the patient a reasonable chance of attaining the goals of a specific therapy.

AUTHORITY FOR WITHDRAWAL OF TREATMENT

Authority for the decision (in order of importance):

1. Request of a decisional patient (see section V, p. 25).
2. Dictates of an advance directive
3. Judgment of guardian or healthcare agent appointed in an advance directive
4. Approval of relatives (spouse, adult children, parents, and adult siblings—in that order; order established by surrogate laws in some states and by convention in others)

5.   Approval of close friends who know the patient's treatment preferences or are able to make decisions that promote the patient's best interest

WITHDRAWAL OF VENTILATORS

1.   **Patients with Brain Death**

When the criteria for brain death have been satisfied (see section XVIII, p. 75), the person is legally dead and there is no obligation to continue ventilation. The ventilator may be removed as soon as the pronouncement of death has been entered into the chart. Organ donation and sensitivity to the family's needs may legitimately delay this procedure for several hours.

2.   **Sentient Patients**

•   **Method of Withdrawal**

When the decision has been made to remove a ventilator from a patient who is (or could be presumed to be) conscious and aware of the consequences, there is no good reason for weaning (the gradual decrease of ventilatory support), as the process often results in dyspnea and a sense of suffocation. After adequate sedation, the ventilator should be discontinued abruptly. Whether the endotracheal tube should be removed or remain in place for suctioning involves a judgment call on the part of the physician.

•   **Sedation**

Before the ventilator is removed, the patient should be sedated heavily with a benzodiazepine or a barbiturate and morphine in doses adequate to produce unconsciousness but not sufficient to produce death. The sedation should be continued until death has occurred. It requires the clinical judgment of the physician at the bedside to know how much and how long to sedate the patient in order to avoid further suffering.

•   **Paralyzing Agents**

Under no circumstances should respiratory paralyzing agents be initiated during ventilator withdrawal, because such

agents hinder evaluation of the patient's suffering and discomfort. However, if a patient is already on these agents, it is
not necessary to wait until the drug is entirely cleared from
the system to begin the process of sedation and ventilator withdrawal.

WITHDRAWAL OF FLUID AND NUTRITION

1. **Patients in a Persistent Vegetative State (PVS)**

    In many states, living will statutes allow persons to state that
    they do not want fluid and nutrition if they are in PVS (see section
    XX, p. 83). Such support can be withdrawn from these patients
    without causing suffering because, by definition, the symptoms of
    thirst and hunger are cortically mediated and cannot be present.

2. **Sentient Patients**
    - **Decision to Withdraw**

        In many states, power of attorney for healthcare laws spe-
        cifically allow a person to give the agent the authority to with-
        hold or to withdraw a feeding tube, regardless of whether the
        patient is in a PVS. The decisional patient, of course, retains
        the right to refuse artificially provided fluid and nutrition.

    - **Effect of Withdrawal**

        When both food and fluid are withdrawn, death usually
        occurs from electrolyte imbalance and dehydration in 10 to
        14 days. If fluid is maintained and food withdrawn, death
        occurs from starvation and may take many weeks. For this
        reason, both food and fluid should be withdrawn or withheld.
        Patients are rarely uncomfortable in the clinical situations in
        which food and fluid are likely to be withdrawn. Ice chips and
        good oral care can assuage symptoms of dry mouth and pro-
        vide comfort care.

    - **Intravenous (IV) Access**

        Occasionally IV access is needed for palliative drug ad-
        ministration. A "keep-open" rate will not provide sufficient
        fluid to prolong the dying process significantly.

FURTHER READING

Rights of the Decisional Patient

The courts have made important statements on the rights of patients to decide about medical treatment. Justice B.N. Cardozo wrote in 1914, "Every human being of adult years and sound mind has a right to determine what shall be done with his own body" (*Schloendorff,* 1914). The *Bartling* decision in California found that "Competent adult patients with serious illnesses which are probably incurable but have not been diagnosed as terminal have the right over the objections of their physicians and the hospital to have life support equipment disconnected despite the fact that withdrawal of such devices will surely hasten death."

Differences between Medical Treatment and Supportive Care

Important differences exist between medical treatment and supportive care. *Medical treatment* is provided by physicians and other health professionals; it is aimed at accomplishing the goals of medical practice. *Supportive care* can be provided by heath professionals but is often provided by other caregivers such as family members; it is aimed at providing comfort to the dying patient. Providing human comfort is imperative, but no "technological imperative" exists. Thus, healthcare professionals are not obligated to provide specialized, life-sustaining treatment to every patient simply because such technology is available.

Difference between Withdrawing and Withholding

The President's Commission for the Study of Ethical Problems in Medicine and Biomedical and Behavioral Research noted in 1983 that the distinction between withholding (failing to initiate) therapy and withdrawing (discontinuing) therapy was not of moral importance. The commission stated that a justification adequate for not commencing a treatment was sufficient for ceasing a treatment that proved ineffective and noted that erecting a higher requirement for cessation might discourage trials of treatments that might sometimes be successful.

Right to Withdrawal of Fluid and Nutrition

Some controversy has existed about whether administration of food and fluid through a feeding tube is a medical treatment or "ordinary care." This has effectively been settled by two court decisions.

In *In re Guardianship of L. W.* (1992), the Wisconsin Supreme Court cited the New Jersey *Conroy* decision (1985), which acknowledged the emotional significance of food but noted that feeding by implanted tubes is a medical procedure with inherent risks and possible side-effects, instituted by skilled healthcare providers to compensate for impaired physical functioning. The court noted that this procedure, analytically, is equivalent to artificial breathing using a respirator.

In an opinion in the US Supreme Court *Cruzan* case (1990), Justice Sandra Day O'Connor said, "Artificial feeding cannot readily be distinguished from other forms of medical treatment. The techniques used to pass food and water into the patient's alimentary tract all involve some degree of intrusion and restraint. Requiring a competent adult to endure such procedures against her will burdens the patient's liberty, dignity and freedom to determine the course of her own treatment."

Effect of Withdrawal of Fluid and Nutrition

Hypernatremia and hypercalcemia occur in many patients after withdrawal of fluid and nutrition. These changes, along with hyperosmolarity, azotemia, and increased endogenous opioids, often produce a sedative effect on the brain during the dying process. Hospice workers have provided other observations:

1. Persons near death often voluntarily stop eating and drinking and do not tolerate substantial volumes of enteral feedings.
2. Dying persons who are given "normal" replacement fluids commonly show signs of fluid overload, including distressing pulmonary edema.
3. Despite substantial physiological deficits, hospice patients almost never report feeling hunger or thirst. Dry mouth and lips are remedied by lubricants and ice chips.
4. Dehydration results in less vomiting and diarrhea, less need to suction secretions, and less dyspnea and peripheral edema.

REFERENCES

American College of Chest Physicians/Society of Critical Care Medicine (ACCP/SCCM) Consensus Panel. Ethical and moral guidelines for the initiation, continuation, and withdrawal of intensive care. *Chest.* 1990;97:949-958.

American Medical Association, Council on Ethical and Judicial Affairs. Decisions near the end of life. *JAMA.* 1992;267:2229-2233.

American Thoracic Society. Withholding and withdrawing life-sustaining therapy. *Ann Intern Med.* 1991;115:478-484.

Bartling v. Superior Court, 209 Cal Rptr 220, 163 Cal App 3d 186 (1984).

Brody H, Campbell ML, Faber-Langendoen K, Ogle KS. Withdrawing intensive life-sustaining treatments: recommendations for a compassionate clinical management. *N Engl J Med.* 1997;336:652-657.

Cruzan v. Director, Missouri Dept of Health, 497 US 261, 111 LEd 2d 224, 110 SCt 2841 (1990).

Hodges MO, Tolle SW. Tube feeding decisions in the elderly. *Clin in Geriatric Med.* 1994;10:475-488.

In re Guardianship of L.W. , 167 Wisc. 2d 53, 482 N.W. 2d 60 (1992).

Katz J. *Experimentation with Human Beings.* New York: Russell Sage Foundation; 1972.

McCann RM, Hall WJ, Groth-Juncker A. Comfort care for terminally ill patients: the appropriate use of nutrition and hydration. *JAMA.* 1994;272:1263-1266.

Meisel A. Legal myths about terminating life support. *Arch Intern Med.* 1991;151:1497-1502.

President's Commission for the Study of Ethical Problems in Medicine and Biomedical Behavioral Research. *Deciding to Forego Life-Sustaining Treatment: Ethical, Medical and Legal Issues in Treatment Decisions.* Washington, DC: US Government Printing Office; 1983.

Printz LA. Terminal dehydration, a compassionate treatment. *Arch Intern Med.* 1992;152:697-700.

Ruark JE, Raffin TA. Initiating and withdrawing life support principles and practice in adult medicine. *N Engl J Med.* 1988;318:25-30.

Schloendorff v. Society of New York Hosp., 211 NY 125, 105 NE 92 (1914).

IV. INFORMED CONSENT

PURPOSE AND DEFINITION

The purpose of the informed consent process is to provide the patient with all of the information necessary to allow a reasonable person to make a prudent treatment choice on his or her own behalf. *Consent* is the patient's voluntary, autonomous authorization to proceed with the proposed intervention.

NURSES' ROLE

It is the nondelegable duty of the physician to obtain informed consent from the patient and to document the process of informed consent. The nurse's role is to validate that the patient has been given the information and to assess whether the patient has additional questions that might require another discussion with the physician. The nurse also may assess the patient's decision-making capacity.

Often a nurse is told to get the patient's signature on the consent form. Nurses must realize, here, that they are not being asked to obtain informed consent from the patient. In cases such as these, the nurse is merely acting as a witness to the identity of the patient and to the patient's signature on the consent form. If a nurse is present at the time the patient signs the consent form, it is a good opportunity for the nurse to assess the patient's level of understanding and to see if the patient wishes further discussion with the physician prior to the proposed intervention.

Some institutions do not use consent forms. At these sites, it is imperative for the physician to adequately document the informed consent process and the patient's agreement to proceed with the proposed intervention. Nurses must be able to locate this documentation in the patient's record and to verbally validate consent with the patient or authorized designee.

ADEQUACY OF INFORMATION

According to the President's Commission for the Study of Ethical Problems in Medicine and Biomedical and Behavioral Research, adequate informed consent requires effort on the part of the physician to ensure comprehension; it involves far more than just a signature on the bottom of a list of possible complications. Such complications can be so overwhelming that patients are unable to appreciate the truly significant information and to make sound decisions.

ELEMENTS OF INFORMED CONSENT

The patient must have a clear understanding of:

1. The disease process (diagnosis in understandable terms)
2. Prognosis
3. Benefits and burdens/risks of recommended treatment
4. Benefits and burdens/risks of reasonable alternative treatments
5. The likely effect of no treatment (which is always an option)

OBTAINING INFORMED CONSENT

Truly informed consent always involves the following elements:

1. Adequate disclosure of information
2. Decisional capacity of the patient
3. Patient's comprehension of the information
4. Voluntariness (freedom from coercion)
5. Consent of the patient

DISCLOSURE STANDARDS USED BY THE COURTS

1. **Professional Community Standard**

   What a capable and reasonable medical practitioner in the same field would reveal to a patient under the same or similar circumstances (about half of the states use this standard).

2. **Reasonable-Patient Standard**

   Because of doubt that a professional community standard can be identified, another standard has been developed, which asks for the information a reasonable patient would consider material to the decision of whether to consent to the procedure offered (the remaining states use this standard).

EXCEPTIONS TO THE INFORMED CONSENT REQUIREMENT

1. **Emergency Privilege**
   - Patient must be unconscious, or without the capacity to make a decision, and no one legally authorized to act as agent for the patient is available.
   - Time must be of the essence, in the sense that there is a risk of serious bodily injury or death.
   - Under the circumstances, a reasonable person would consent.

2. **Therapeutic Privilege Disclosure Would Have an Adverse Effect on the Patient's Health**
   - The physician must take into account the circumstances of the patient.
   - The physician must believe that a full disclosure of the information will have a significantly adverse impact on the patient.
   - This standard has been much abused in the past. It should be used infrequently and with great discretion.

3. **Patient Does Not Have Decisional Capacity**
   Patient must be decisional in order for consent to be informed and voluntary.

4. **Waiver of Rights**
   Patient does not desire to have information. The physician, in these instances, should not force the issue but should document it well and ask for permission to inform a surrogate. The nurse may assist here by locating a surrogate decision maker.

5. **Disagreement with Decision Maker in Lifesaving Situations**
   Sometimes a physician believes that he or she must act against the wishes of a patient's husband, wife, or parent(s) if the physician believes that person's decision to treat, or usually not to treat, is not in the best interest of the patient. In these cases, the physician seeks a court order to treat against the will of the decision maker. For example, when a child needs a blood transfusion and the parents are Jehovah's Witnesses and refuse to allow the transfusion, physicians may seek a court order to allow the transfusion.

HOW LONG IS CONSENT GOOD?

Consent forms are usually dated, but sometimes the patient may grant consent in the physician's office weeks in advance of the proposed intervention. *Is it acceptable to use a consent form that has been obtained in advance?* Because many healthcare institutions have policies addressing this issue and some states have laws or regulations that must be followed, nurses must be familiar with and act in accordance with the policies/regulations of the organization and state where they practice. However, if there is no specific policy that addresses a length of time or expiration date for a consent form, the answer to the question above a qualified "yes." Of course, the qualifier is that the patient's condition under which the original consent was signed has not changed. For example, if a patient agrees to surgery 2 months before the scheduled procedure, and in the time between the signing of the consent form and the surgical intervention the patient experiences a heart attack, then the conditions (especially the risks and benefits) may have drastically changed, which could invalidate the consent. In such cases, the physician must reevaluate the patient and help the patient to make another decision relative to the patient's current condition.

REFERENCES

Brody H. Transparency: informed consent in primary care. *Hastings Cent Rep*. 1989; 19(5):5-9.

Gilmore PD. An ethical perspective. Waiver of informed consent requirements in certain medical emergencies: ethical dilemmas. *J Nurs Law,* 1997;4(2):23-39.

Meisel A, Kuczewski M. Legal and ethical myths about informed consent. *Arch Intern Med*. 1996;156:2521-2526.

President's Commission for the Study of Ethical Problems in Medicine and Biomedical and Behavioral Research. *Making Health Care Decisions: The Ethical and Legal Implications of Informed Consent in the Patient-Physician Relationship*. Washington, DC: US Government Printing Office; 1982.

V. COMPETENCE AND DECISION-MAKING CAPACITY

DEFINITIONS
1. **Competence**

   Competence and *incompetence* are legal terms. Technically, a patient remains competent until a court says otherwise.
2. **Decision-Making Capacity**

   The determination of decision-making capacity can be made by medical personnel and does not require a court hearing.

NURSES' ROLE
Because nurses are the primary caregivers in most healthcare institutions, it falls within the realm of nursing practice to assess decision-making capacity. The nurse can assist the medical team by providing an evaluative opinion regarding the patient's ability to make decisions. The nurse is constantly assessing the patient's capacity as a part of daily patient care. As the patient's mental status changes, the nurse is often the first to notice. The nurse must relay the information to the physician as soon as possible when issues of decisionality are at stake.

CLINICAL ASSESSMENT OF DECISION-MAKING CAPACITY
In assessing a patient's ability to make autonomous judgments, one must evaluate the three distinct aspects of decision-making capacity:
1. **Ability to Understand**
   - The ability to comprehend the given information about diagnosis and treatment and to identify the issue at hand (To test this, ask the patient to paraphrase the discussion.)
   - The ability to appreciate the impact of the disease and its consequences (To test this, ask the patient to state the major options and the most likely outcome for each option.)
2. **Ability to Evaluate**
   - The ability to deliberate in accordance with one's own values

- The ability to manipulate information rationally and to compare risks and benefits of the options
- The ability to make choices that are not irrational and to give the reasons for them
- The ability to maintain a consistent choice over time

3. **Ability to Communicate**
   - The ability to communicate choices (To test this, ask the patient to state his or her choice of treatment options.)

If the patient demonstrates satisfactory responses in all three areas, he or she is said to have "decision-making capacity," to be "decisional," or to be "capacitated."

SLIDING SCALE OF DECISION-MAKING CAPACITY

1. If there is a favorable expectation from the patient's choice (little risk, large benefit), then a relatively low level of decision-making capacity is required.
2. If there is a balance of risk and benefit from the patient's choice, then a moderate level of decision-making capacity is required.
3. If expectations from the patient's choice are not favorable (great risk with little chance of benefit), then a high level of decision-making capacity is necessary.

THE MATURE MINOR

By legal definition, minors (under the age of 18 in most states) are not competent to make major healthcare decisions. Many states give minors limited autonomy; they are specifically allowed to obtain contraception, abortion, and treatment for venereal disease or substance abuse without parental permission. In many states, minors who are married or living independently and supporting themselves are considered to be "emancipated minors" and competent to make their own healthcare decisions. Moreover, developing case law on the "mature minor" now recognizes that, as the adolescent's age increases toward maturity, he or she should have a progressively greater part in the decision-making process.

DECISION MAKING FOR INCAPACITATED PATIENTS

When a surrogate acts for an incapacitated patient, the basis for decision is one of the following:

1. **Substituted Judgment**

   This is the guideline the surrogate should use if the patient has expressed a preference before becoming incompetent, or if the surrogate knows the patient well enough to determine what the patient would choose if he or she were still decisional.

2. **Best Interest**

   This is the standard the surrogate must use when he or she has no clear idea of what the patient might choose. It is what a reasonable person might choose in the same context and is based on what is ultimately best for this particular patient in these particular circumstances.

   When a patient has a legal guardian, this individual has the right to refuse life-sustaining treatment based on the patient's best interest in the light of the diagnosis, prognosis, and medical goals of treatment.

DIFFICULTIES IN MAKING JUDGMENTS FOR THE INCAPACITATED PATIENT

There are several complications in making ethical decisions that are in the best interest of an incapacitated patient.

1. We do not know the wishes of the patient in regard to the withdrawal of life-sustaining treatment in the context of the immediate clinical situation.

2. Since we do not have the autonomous wishes of the incompetent patient to act upon, we must rely on surrogates and professionals to make these decisions.

3. It is preferable to make quality-of-life judgments based on the patient's own assessment. Because incompetent patients cannot provide this information, quality-of-life determinations become subjective on the part of others—a risky evaluation at best.

REFERENCES

Cohen LM, McCue JD, Green GM. Do clinical and formal assessments of the capacity of patients in the intensive care unit to make decisions agree? *Arch Intern Med.* 1993;153;2481-2485.

Drane JF. Competency to give informed consent: a model for making clinical assessments. *JAMA.* 1984;252:925-927.

Emanuel EJ. What criteria should guide decision makers for incompetent patients? *Lancet.* 1988;1:170-171.

Miles SH, Koepp R, Weber EP. Advance end-of-life treatment planning. *Arch Intern Med.* 1996;156:1062-1068.

Schneiderman LJ, Arras, JD. Counseling patients to counsel physicians on future care in the event of patient incompetence. *Ann Intern Med.* 1985;102:693-698.

VI. CONFIDENTIALITY

ANA *CODE OF ETHICS FOR NURSES*

According to the American Nurses Association (ANA) *Code of Ethics for Nurses with Interpretive Statements*, the nurse safeguards the patient's right to privacy by judiciously protecting information of a confidential nature.

The patient's confidence that information given to the nurse will remain private is an important element in the nurse-patient relationship. Without such assurance, the patient might be unwilling to divulge information critical to his or her care.

BASIS FOR THE PRINCIPLE

1. Inherent respect for an individual's privacy and autonomy
2. Special trust inherent in the nurse-patient relationship
3. The good of society
4. Prevention of harm to the patient

EXCEPTIONS

There may be legal exceptions to the nurse's duty to maintain confidentiality that necessitate divulgence. Among these are:

1. Testifying in court
2. Reporting communicable disease
3. Reporting child abuse, spouse abuse, or elder abuse
4. Reporting gunshot or suspicious wounds if there is a reasonable cause to believe that the wound occurred as a result of a crime
5. Reporting for workers' compensation cases

BREACH OF CONFIDENTIALITY

There may be situations in which there is an ethical demand for the nurse to consider breaching patient confidentiality. Such a problem may occur when a patient who is HIV positive refuses to tell his or her spouse or significant other of the infection, thus placing the other at risk of contracting a lethal disease. The nurse who is aware of this is in a bind between duty to the patient and the stronger ethical demand to warn an unsuspecting person of significant danger. Such a breach is justified when all of the following conditions apply:

1. A high probability exists of serious physical harm to a person.
2. A likely benefit will result from breaking the confidence (for example, the harm can be prevented).
3. The breach is a last resort; persuasion and other approaches have failed.
4. The breach is generalizable; it would be reasonable for a nurse or doctor to breach your confidence and to treat you in the same way if you were the patient.

As more and more patient records are maintained electronically, it has become more difficult for healthcare providers to ensure confidentiality of patient records. Organizations are requiring nurses to sign agreements of confidentiality when it comes to computer passwords and codes. It has never been acceptable practice to leave a patient's chart out and open in a public area, but today a nurse must be careful not to allow patient information to be publicly visible from a computer screen. The best method to promote confidentiality is to require authorized staff to log off whenever they have finished reviewing or documenting patient information at a computer terminal.

REFERENCES

American Nurses Association. *Code of Ethics for Nurses with Interpretive Statements*. Kansas City, Mo: American Nurses Association; 2001.<http://www.ana.org/ethics/#3>.

Brennan TA. AIDS and the limits of confidentiality: the physician's duty to warn contacts of seropositive individuals. *J Gen Intern Med*. 1989;4:242-246.

Gostin LO et al. Privacy and security of personal information in a new health care system. *JAMA* 1993;270:2487-2493.

Health and Public Policy Committee of the American College of Physicians and Infectious Diseases Society of America. Acquired immunodeficiency syndrome. *Ann Intern Med*. 1986;104:575-581.

VII. ADVOCACY

DEFINITION

Advocacy describes the act of pleading for, supporting, urging by argument, recommending publicly, and espousing actively. Illness can affect the patient's autonomy and ability to make decisions, which places the nurse in a powerful position. Because the patient is perceived as extremely vulnerable in the healthcare setting, the role of the nurse as advocate has become very important to patient care.

IMPLICATIONS FOR NURSES

As patient advocates, nurses accept responsibility to safeguard the rights of patients and to ensure both the quality and continuity of patient care. The nurse continually assesses the care of the patient and works to ensure that the patient's physical, emotional, and ethical needs are met. The nurse, as a moral agent of the patient, must be ready and able to advocate for the patient's needs whenever necessary while providing care.

In the discipline of nursing, advocacy is often viewed as a duty or obligation that arises from the nurse's role as continual observer of the patient's condition. The American Hospital Association's "A Patient's Bill of Rights" lists advocacy as one of the rights of patients, and it declares that "activities must be conducted with an overriding concern for the patient, and above all, the recognition of his dignity as a human being."

The nurse's role as a patient advocate has been described as having three basic components:

1. Informing patients of their rights in a particular situation
2. Ensuring that patients are given all the information they require to make an informed decision
3. Supporting patients in decisions they make

As a patient advocate, the nurse is responsible for safeguarding the patient from the incompetence of other healthcare professionals. This may be a statutory duty as well as an ethical one.

WHO MUST ADVOCATE FOR PATIENTS?

All healthcare providers should function as patient advocates. Nurses, however, are in a position of consistent closeness and accessibility to patients. Nurses are often available to hear patient concerns and discuss such issues with the patient, and consequently, nurses often become the mediator or messenger in relaying patient concerns to other appropriate members of the healthcare team.

Nurses have the potential to develop relationships with patients that put them in a position of trust. Patients trust that nurses will support and follow through with any concerns or issues that have been discussed. Nurses may, at times, become sounding boards for their patients, encouraging them and providing opportunities to discuss their concerns with their physicians or family members. This support can be classified as advocacy.

Nursing is based on a therapeutic and caring relationship. Nurses are encouraged to stay within the parameters that define a professional and therapeutic relationship between nurse and the patient/family, although they often receive little guidance about how to do so. For example, in cases involving a pediatric patient whose parents are making decisions and identifying the child's needs, the nurse may have difficulty determining whether to advocate for the pediatric patient or for the child's parents. An unclear therapeutic relationship can undermine nurses' advocacy efforts.

UNDERSTANDING ADVOCACY AS ETHICAL PRACTICE

Are advocacy and empowerment dichotomous or synchronous concepts? If advocacy is an expectation of the nurse's role, then nurses should have a certain amount of authority inherent in the role to ensure that patients' needs are met. However, nurses experience frustration when they attempt to function in the role of patient advocate. Conflicts may be resolved more quickly if the nurse has authority to confront the situation when it first presents. Healthcare administrators must ensure that nurses are given a voice to advocate for their patients. Corporate compliance is one way in which organizations are attempting to promote advocacy in healthcare, especially via nurses.

Additionally, there is often confusion between the nurse's responsibility to support the patient and the institution, and the nurse's ability to support his or her own moral stance. Nurses must act according to their values as well as their practice standards and code of ethics. In addition to advocating for patients, nurses should advocate for themselves if they are put in a situation that requires compromising their personal values. Nurses must recognize when they must "opt out" of certain aspects of patient care that are in conflict with their religious or moral beliefs. Nurses should discuss this issue when interviewing for a position, because not all nursing roles allow for such opportunity to step back from providing care (see section X, p. 45).

ADVOCACY VERSUS WHISTLEBLOWING

The term *whistleblowing* has a negative connotation, and the nurse who blows the whistle on an organization, practice, or individual may not be viewed as a hero or heroine but rather as a "squealer" or "stool pigeon." Whistleblowing can be a means to an end, and, if viewed positively, can be viewed as another form of advocacy. The ultimate goal is to facilitate communication and obtain a constructive solution. The following factors apply to whistleblowing:

1. The issue must be serious.
2. The individual must have capacity or competence to judge the seriousness of the issue and should verify the issue. In essence, a nurse can make a judgment about improper nursing practice, but not necessarily about medical practice.
3. The individual must exhaust all internal options first.

GUIDELINES FOR WHISTLEBLOWING

Focus on the disclosure about the issue itself —*not* on the personalities or the politics of those involved. Write a summary or report of what happened. Document what actions were taken. Send a copy to management, and save the documentation. Use internal channels first. Anticipate and document any retaliation. Follow these steps:

1. Identify issue.
    *   Establish a database.

- Verify facts.
- Document.
- Have a legitimate case.
- Be prepared to go on record because anonymous disclosure is less convincing.

2. Plan.
- Plan strategies.
- Obtain support.
- Outline an action plan.
- Work within the chain of command.

3. Implement.
- Contact the supervisor and follow the institutional chain of command.
- Use internal channels.
- Keep a record.
- Identify deadlines.
- Contact regulatory or professional agencies.
- Contact the media only as a last resort.

BECOMING AN ADVOCATE

Assuming that the stance of a patient advocate involves acting on ethical principles and values, nurses in all areas of practice must be prepared to identify issues of advocacy and take action as needed. The nurse-patient relationship allows nurses to advocate for their patients as well as for themselves. Nurses can empower their patients by providing opportunities for patients to make autonomous decisions about healthcare and by educating patients about appropriate administrative protocols (such as patients' rights and hospital policies and procedures that will best meet the individual patient's needs). The keys to advocacy include the following:

1. Understanding advocacy as an ethical concept
2. Understanding advocacy and its relationship to nursing practice

3. Analyzing personal communication skills and developing them as needed
4. Identifying situations where advocacy is necessary
5. Taking action (advocating for patients)

REFERENCES

American Hospital Association. A patient's bill of rights. In Reich RT, ed. *Encyclopedia of Bioethics*. New York: Free Press, 1978;4:1782-1783.

Court case. Blowing the whistle. *Nurs.* 2000;30(4):28.

Fry ST. *Ethics in Nursing Practice: A Guide to Ethical Decision Making*. Geneva: International Council of Nurses; 1994.

Kohnke A. The nurse as advocate. *Am J Nurs.* 1980;80:2038-2039.

Liaschenko J. Ethics in the work of acting for patients. *Advances in Nurs Sci.* 1995;18:1-12.

Martin GW. Communication breakdown or ideal speech situation: the problem of nurse advocacy. *Nurs Ethics.* 1998;2:147-157.

McDonald S, Ahern K. The professional consequences of whistleblowing by nurses. *J Prof Nurs.* 2000;16(6):313-21.

Salladay SA. Ethical problems. Whistle blowing: going public: risky move? *Nurs.* 1997;27(5):68.

Schroeter K. Ethical perception and resulting action in perioperative nurses. *AORN J.* 1999;5:991-1002.

Sloan AJ. Legally speaking. Whistleblowing: there are risks! *RN.* 1999;62(7):65-68.

Sloan AJ. Whistleblowing and patient advocacy: do the right thing... but do it right. *Virginia Nurses Today.* 1997;5(3):14-5.

Snowball J. Asking nurses about advocating for patients: 'reactive' and 'proactive' accounts. *J Adv Nurs.* 1996;24: 67-75.

"Whistleblower" advocates for protection of nurses who fight unsafe conditions. *Mass Nurse.* 1997;67(4):1.

Wilmot S. Nurses and whistleblowing: the ethical issues. *J Adv Nurs.* 2000;32(5):1051-7.

VIII. LEGAL ISSUES

INTRODUCTION

In many ethical issues in nursing, legal issues may also arise. Ethics and law both set norms or standards for conduct. Law often expresses a minimal ethical societal consensus—one that society is willing to enforce through civil judgments or criminal sanctions. However, there are areas of conduct that the law does not and cannot address. Many areas of human conduct, including the nurse-patient relationship, are governed by ethical behavior but not mandated by law. Nonetheless, in considering ethical issues in nursing practice, the law has been and continues to be an important consideration.

Occasionally, the best ethical course of action may appear to conflict with legal understanding. In these cases, consultation from the ethics committee and risk management may be helpful in resolving this dilemma.

US LAW

In the United States, law is created in one of two systems—federal and state. It is made by judges (common law), legislatures (statutory law), and executive agencies empowered by legislatures (regulatory law). The law's methods of enforcement are either civil (most commonly, monetary judgments) or criminal (fines and/or prison). End-of-life legal issues have generally been resolved through state civil common law and state civil statutory law. Each system of common law (federal and state) has its own appellate process where cases may be appealed and resolved by an intermediate appellate court or, ultimately, a supreme court. These appellate court decisions are mandatory precedent for lower courts in their jurisdiction. These decisions may also be persuasive for courts in other jurisdictions.

Although federal legislative law and US Supreme Court decisions apply to all jurisdictions in the United States, each state's legislature and state supreme court also make law within the constraints of federal law. Generally, there are common themes that run through these laws, although particular state laws have some variations. Some of the most important legal principles in clinical ethics are widely accepted among the states, but it is important for nurses to become familiar with their state's statutes and cases on ethical issues and to understand how state law varies on these themes.

10 IMPORTANT PRINCIPLES IN CASE AND STATUTORY LAW

1. **Nurses have a legal duty to act in the patient's best interest.**

   This duty, known as a fiduciary duty, requires the nurse to act in the patient's best interest. This duty is legally enforceable, but is dependent upon the patient's (or guardian's) permission to care for the patient.

2. **Patients must give informed consent for testing, procedures, treatment, and research.**

   For example, in *Canterbury* (1972), a patient's guardian was not informed of the risk of paralysis for spinal surgery, which a reasonable patient would have found material in a decision on whether to undergo the surgery. The Federal District Court in Washington, DC, held that the patient's guardian should have been informed. About half of jurisdictions hold that the standard should be information that a reasonable patient would want to know, while the others hold that the standard should be what the prudent professional should disclose.

3. **Patients who have the capacity to refuse treatment should be informed of the consequences of the refusal.**

   For example, in *Truman* (1980), a patient who refused pap smears during her physical exams later developed cervical cancer and died. The California Supreme Court held that the patient should have been informed of the nature of the proposed test and the consequences of her refusal. Decisional patients who refuse treatment may not always be willing to hear the consequences of their refusal, but it should be offered. In the case of a life- or limb-threatening emergency, if the patient does not have decision-making capacity and no one is available who is legally authorized to make healthcare decisions for the patient, the patient may not be able to refuse treatment.

4. **Adult patients with decision-making capacity may refuse treatment, including life-sustaining medical treatment.**

    This refusal is not suicide, and complying with this refusal is not homicide.

    For example, in *Bouvia* (1986), a patient with cerebral palsy and quadriplegia who had decision-making capacity (and was not suicidal) refused artificial fluid and nutrition, even though it was thought that she would die without the treatment. The California Appellate court held that she could forgo the treatment. The US Supreme Court in *Cruzan* (1990) has upheld the decisional patient's right to refuse life-sustaining medical treatment.

5. **Adult patients who become incapacitated retain the right to refuse treatment, which may be expressed through an advance directive or through other evidence of the patient's wishes.**

    For example, in *Cruzan* (1990), the parents of a woman who was in a persistent vegetative state (PVS) asked to have artificial nutrition and hydration withdrawn. The US Supreme Court stated that the adult decisional patient can refuse life-sustaining medical treatment and that this right can be asserted by a legal representative of the patient, such as a guardian or healthcare agent.

6. **The state may require clear evidence of the adult incapacitated patient's wishes to refuse life-sustaining medical treatment.**

    For example, in *Cruzan,* the US Supreme Court held that the right of the now-nondecisional patient to forgo life-sustaining medical treatment may be restricted by a state's requirement for clear evidence of the patient's wishes, such as an advance directive, such as a living will or power of attorney for healthcare.

7. **Decisions for a child should be made according to the child's best interest.**

    In general, parents are assumed to act in the child's best interest, but, on occasion, parents may refuse treatments or choose inappropriate treatment for their child. Courts routinely override parents' decisions when it is judged that the treatment for a life-threatening condition will be effective and without serious risks or side-effects. In cases of handicapped infants, the federal Child Abuse Amendments of 1984 and subsequent regulations, known as "Baby Doe" regulations, may limit the circumstances under which life-sustaining treatment may be withheld.

8. **Adolescents may be able to make certain healthcare decisions for themselves.**

Many states recognize that adolescents can make certain health-care decisions for themselves such as treatment for sexually transmitted diseases or drug and alcohol abuse. These exceptions are most frequently expressed:

- In statutes that enable such decision making for specific diseases
- In statutes that enable adolescents who meet certain criteria to be recognized as emancipated minors
- By courts that may find certain adolescents mature enough to make these decisions

9. **Healthcare providers have a legal duty to keep patient information confidential.**

For example, in *Humphers* (1985), the Oregon Supreme Court held that disclosing a patient's identity to the daughter whom she had given up for adoption was a violation of the duty to keep the patient's confidence. In general, states have statutes that delineate who may have access to medical information about a patient and under what circumstances.

10. **This legal duty of confidentiality may be breached by an overriding duty to protect others who are endangered by the patient.**

For example, in *Tarasoff* (1976), the California Supreme Court found that, despite a duty of confidentiality, a patient who poses a danger to another may give rise to a countervailing duty to breach the confidentiality in order to protect the other person.

REFERENCES

Bouvia v. Superior Court (Glenchur), 179 CalApp3d 1127, 225 CalRptr 297 (2nd Dist 1986).

Canterbury v. Spence, 464 F2d 772 (DC Cir 1972).

Cruzan v. Director, Missouri Department of Health, 497 US 261, 110 SCt 2841 (1990).

Humphers v. First Interstate Bank of Oregon, 298 Ore 706, 696 P2nd 527 (1985).

Meisel A. Legal myths about terminating life support. *Arch Intern Med.* 1991;1551:1497-1502.

Tarasoff v. Regents of the Univ of Cal, 17 Cal3d 425, 131 CalRptr 14, 551 P2d 334 (1976).

Truman v. Thomas, 27 Cal3d 285, 165 CalRptr 308, 611 P2d 902 (1980).

IX. PEDIATRIC NURSING ISSUES

STANDARDS: BEST INTEREST VERSUS SUBSTITUTED JUDGMENT

Pediatric decision making begins with trying to determine what is best for the child.

One of the most difficult aspects of making decisions regarding the treatment of children is knowing what this is. Parents should be involved in this process. Most minors (children or adolescents under the age of 18) are, by law, unable to give consent or refusal to treatment. Unlike adults, pediatric patients have never possessed decision-making capacity, although some children who are "mature minors" are legally able to consent to or refuse treatment, and can be treated like adults. Nonetheless, this is the appropriate standard for decision making. In most cases, medical decision making ultimately rests in the hands of the parents or guardians, with guidance from healthcare providers. This does not mean that the viewpoints of children, and especially adolescents, should not be considered in decisions about treatment.

THE NURSE AS CHILD ADVOCATE

In pediatrics, one of the primary roles of nurses and physicians is that of child advocate. Reasonable medical measures that are in the best interest of the child should be employed, with at least a trial of treatment even in the most critically ill children. As in adult medicine, futility may be a contraindication to continued treatment in some cases.

It is imperative for the nurse to advocate for the child's preferences when appropriate. The nurse must know that parental power is not absolute and is restricted by the welfare of the child. The nurse must be able to demonstrate age-specific competence in the care of children of different ages. An adolescent or mature minor, for example, may be able to offer much more participation in assenting to treatment decisions.

THE NURSE AS PARENT ADVOCATE

As advisors to the parents of their patients, pediatricians and pediatric nurses can counsel and support parents as they reach decisions regarding the best interest of their child (see section IV, pg. 21).

This is a difficult process, for clinicians must be as objective as possible in giving an opinion or medical recommendation. Healthcare providers may fail in the role of advisor in two ways. They may hide behind the "objectivity" of the medical facts and fail to give any guidance on what is medically and ethically correct, merely saying, "These are the options. What do you want me to do?" Conversely, they may knowingly or unknowingly manipulate the parents into making the decision that the healthcare team prefers by relating only those facts that would support a particular decision.

It is useful to give the parents time and to encourage them to get a second or even a third opinion in difficult circumstances. If the ethical conflict persists, a consultation with the ethics committee may be appropriate.

NEONATAL INTENSIVE CARE

Before our current neonatal technology became available, medical care for critically ill newborns was mainly supportive care. Data collected in the neonatal intensive care unit (NICU) confirm that infants with increasingly low birth weights are surviving. In the 1960s, the smallest infants for whom we could provide ventilatory support weighed 1500 grams; with the advent of new technology, 500-gram infants can now be maintained on ventilatory support.

This success, however, is not unqualified. Ventilatory management has been difficult, and multiple complications may occur. The low-birth-weight neonate may have patent ductus arteriosus, immature brain and germinal matrix, and incomplete retinal vascularization. Although some low-birth-weight infants grow and develop normally despite the challenges of prematurity, others have chronic physical and developmental disabilities. It is extremely difficulty to predict reliably an individual child's long-term prognosis. The practice of aggressive treatment and resuscitation of infants in the NICU raises a number of ethical questions.

In addition, heightened public awareness and resulting increases in funding for neonatal intensive care technology, while inarguably benefiting some infants, may also have the unintended effect of diverting attention and funding from basic prenatal care. As is true in adult medicine, the recent focus on high technology is threatening the traditional primary care focus of pediatrics.

ETHICAL ISSUES

1. Neonatal ethical issues focus on the aggressiveness of treatment and resuscitation of infants who are already being treated aggressively in the NICU.
2. Pediatric ethics issues for the mature minor mirror those of the adult patient. The capacity of children to be involved in decisions depends upon their age and intellectual capacity.

PEDIATRIC PAIN MANAGEMENT

Historically, pediatric pain has been undertreated, partly because of a persistent myth that children do not experience pain in the same way that adults do. We now know that this belief is untrue, but it has only been since the 1980s that pain in children has been aggressively treated. Some clinicians still undertreat pain today out of concern that opioids may cause respiratory depression. However, this phenomenon is extremely uncommon if small doses are used and titrated to effect.

One of the most difficult aspects of pain management in children is accurate assessment of the severity of the pain, particularly in preverbal children. Behavioral assessment tools are often used for younger children, but visual scales should be used whenever possible in older children. Distraction techniques and parental presence may also be of help.

Nursing staff should be familiar with the age-specific care of children (such as pediatric airway/cardiovascular physiology, pharmacology, and behavioral and emotional responses of pediatric patients). In addition, nurses should be aware that inadequate pain control may result in hypertension, prolonged recovery time, and emotional distress. To be ethical and compassionate, healthcare providers are obligated to become educated about pediatric pain issues.

ETHICAL NURSING PRACTICE

The pediatric nurse must be knowledgeable regarding the age-specific needs of pediatric patients. It is the nurse's responsibility to recognize and respect aspects of pain management that are unique to children. The nurse in this role becomes the parental surrogate, advocating for the child, assessing pain, and providing timely and effective relief. Understanding pain management across the life span is an integral part of ethical nursing practice.

REFERENCES

American Nurses Association. ANA code for nurses with interpretive statements. *Mass Nurse.* 1997;9:4-6.

Bleich JD. The ethics of pain management. *Cancer Invest* 1994;12:362-363.

Cauldwell, CB. Induction, maintenance, and emergence. In: Gregory GA, ed. *Pediatric Anesthesia.* 3rd ed. New York: Churchill Livingstone; 1995;227,792.

Graves SA, Berman LS. Caring for the child in a general postanesthesia care unit. *Am J Anesthesiol.* 1996;23:176-181.

Hall SC. Pediatric postanesthesia recovery care. *J Clin Anesth.* 1995;7:600-605.

Harrison H. Principles for family centered neonatal care. *Pediatrics.* 1993;92:643-650.

Hefferman P, Heilig S. Giving "moral distress" a voice: ethical concerns among neonatal intensive care unit personnel. *Cambridge Q Healthcare Ethics.* Spring 1999;8(2):173-178.

Joint Commission on Accreditation of Healthcare Organizations. *Accreditation Manual for Hospitals,* Chicago: JCAHO; 1995:1 (HR.3, HR.3.2, HR.4).

Jonsen AR, Siegler M, Winslade WJ. *Clinical Ethics.* 3rd ed. New York: McGraw-Hill; 1992.

Kachoyeanos MK, Zollo MB. Ethics in pain management of infants and children. *American Journal of Maternal Child Nursing,* 1995;20:142-147.

Kobs A. Competence: the shot heard around the nursing world. *Nurs Manage.* 1997;2:10,12-13.

Lantos JD, et al. Providing and forgoing resuscitative therapy for babies of very low birth weight. *J Clin Ethics.* 1992;3:283-287.

Lee B, Wheeler T. Emergence and recovery from anesthesia for pediatric patients in the postanesthesia care unit. *Pediatr Ann.* 1997;8:461-469.

McDaniel C. Enhancing nurses' ethical practice. *Nurs Clin North Am.* 1998;2:299-311.

President's Commission for the Study of Ethical Problems in Medicine and Biomedical and Behavioral Research. *Deciding to Forego Life-Sustaining Treatment.* Washington, DC: US Government Printing Office; 1983.

Rushton, CH. Child/family advocacy: ethical issues, practical strategies. *Crit Care,* 1993;21:S387-S388.

Speers AT, Ziolkowski L. Preparing for the future: perianesthesia orientation. *J Perianesthesia Nurs.* 1996;3:133-142.

X. OBSTETRIC NURSING ISSUES

ETHICAL ISSUES

Ethical issues in obstetric/gynecologic (OB/GYN) nursing are different from those faced in other nursing specialties in that the focus is usually on two individuals, the mother and the unborn baby. Often decisions have their basis in personal values that stem from religious, social, and/or cultural beliefs. According to Lo (2000), issues in OB/GYN ethics are different from ethics issues faced in other specialties because:

1. They involve philosophical questions that science cannot resolve.
2. Two patients are involved.
3. Although decisions are very personal, third parties seek to gain influence.
4. New reproductive technologies raise unprecedented dilemmas.

ETHICS ISSUES SPECIFIC TO OB/GYN NURSING

1. Emergencies (life and limb)
2. Prenatal testing (such as testing for HIV, genetic testing)
3. Adolescents and reproduction
4. Consent
5. Family planning
6. Sterilization
7. Substance abuse during pregnancy
8. Student participation in pelvic exams
9. Cesarean section upon maternal request

ISSUES OF CONSCIENCE

If a nurse has a belief that conflicts with his or her ability to perform some nursing function or duty, the nurse is responsible for notifying the employing agency so that a staff accommodation can be made, if possible. Nurses' requests, however, cannot result in abandoning patients or burdening other nurses or ancillary personnel in the department. Nurses and employers should take a proactive approach to situations involving potential conflict.

1. The nurse should discuss the potential for conflict before accepting employment in a healthcare setting.
2. The employer should anticipate potential conflicts around the patient populations cared for by the agency and develop guidelines addressing the potential conflicts.
3. The nurse may need to make a career change if an area of nursing is not conducive to her or his moral or religious beliefs and values.

REFERENCES

Chervenak FA, McCullough LB. Ethics in obstetrics and gynecology: an overview. *Eur Journal of Obstet, Gynecol & Reprod Biol.* 1997;75:91-94.

Chervenak FA, McCullough LB. Obstetric ethics and the abortion controversy. *Am J Ethics & Med.* 1994;3(1):3-6.

Chervenak FA, McCullough LB. What is obstetric ethics? *J Perinat Med.* 1995;23:331-341.

Ethical issues in obstetric-gynecologic education. ACOG Committee Opinion No. 181, April 1997. *Int J Gynaecol Obstet.* 1997;57:327-330.

Ethical issues in pregnancy counseling: a guide to counseling prospective parents in light of current capabilities for evaluation of pregnancy outcome, as well as obstetric management. ACOG Committee Opinion No. 61, March 1998, p. 1.

Lo B. *Resolving Ethical Dilemmas: A Guide for Clinicians.* Baltimore: Williams & Wilkins; 2000:302-309.

Proimos J. Confidentiality issues in the adolescent population. *Curr Opin Pediatr.* 1997;9:325-328.

Tranquilli A, et al. A new ethical and clinical dilemma in obstetric practice: cesarean section "on maternal request" [letter and response]. *Am J Obstet Gynecol.* 1997 1997 1997;177:245-246.

XI. PSYCHIATRIC NURSING ISSUES

DECISION-MAKING CAPACITY

A psychiatric diagnosis, *per se*, does not imply that a patient lacks the capacity to make an informed decision about treatment. A decisional patient's refusal should be respected if attempts at persuasion are unsuccessful. Additionally, patients who are involuntarily committed may still be deemed competent to refuse psychiatric treatment. Because decisional capacity is determined with regard to specific tasks, a patient who is not decisional in regard to refusal of commitment may still be deemed competent to refuse medications or procedures. Some consider it pointless to withhold from severely impaired patients the very treatments that are likely to restore their autonomy. In this view, Lo asserts that short-term involuntary treatment, which may improve the underlying psychiatric illness, is a lesser infringement on the patient's freedom than prolonged involuntary hospitalization without treatment.

Of greatest concern in regard to the psychiatric patient is the potential for impaired cognitive functioning related to his or her illness. This is especially true when assessing the patient's ability to consent to procedures or participation in research protocols. Nurses must be aware that psychiatric patients may be:

1. Unable to make informed decisions
2. Unable to care for themselves
3. Unable to know right from wrong
4. Unable to control their impulses
5. Not legally or morally responsible for their actions

RESEARCH ISSUES

Psychiatric patients are considered a vulnerable population. Although they may be able to make some decisions related to activities of daily living, they are often unable to decide such involved issues as participation in research. Because family members of such patients may be desperate for adequate/effective treatment, they may not be able to consent freely in all cases.

Researchers must take care not to be coercive in obtaining consent.

When research is conducted on a psychiatric unit, nurses must be alert to ethical issues of coercion and consent.

1. Patients may be easily motivated to remain in a study by offers of cigarettes or privileges.
2. Patients may not understand their right of refusal to participate.
3. Patients who have been involuntarily committed may need to obtain research consent from guardians.
4. Family members or significant others should be involved in the discussion about consent to participate in research.

IMPLICATIONS FOR NURSES

Nurses in psychiatric practice are truly in the role of patient advocate and must strive to help their patients communicate their wishes about treatment. Patients may also talk with nurses about end-of-life issues and may request an advance directive. If a patient is not consistently decisional, it may be difficult to write an advance directive. However, if the patient has demonstrated some consistency of thought or has made similar requests over a period of time, this is often a sign of their wishes.

Written informed consent is required for the administration of psychotropic medications, unless there is an emergency situation in which the patient presents as a danger to self or others.

Nurses also have a duty to protect third parties from harm. Although confidentiality is important in the nurse-patient relationship, "the protective privilege ends where the public peril begins" (*Tarasoff*). Thus, if a nurse thinks that a patient is harmful to himself or others, the assessment must be reported to the psychiatrist and any others in accordance with institutional policy and state or federal law.

REFERENCES

Clark A, Barker P, Glover D. Dilemmas: Is it right to collude in a patient's delusion? *Nurs Times* 2000;96(22):1-7.
Idziak JM. *Ethical Dilemmas in Allied Health*. Dubuque, Iowa: Simon and Kolz; 2000.
Lo B. *Resolving Ethical Dilemmas: A Guide for Clinicians*. Baltimore: Williams & Wilkins; 2000.
Tarasoff v Regents of the University of California, 551 P2d 334 (Cal 1976).
Twomey JG. Ethical voices of pediatric mental health nurses. *J Pediatr Nurs*. 2000;15(1):36-46.

XII. THE DIFFICULT PATIENT

Some patients are very difficult to care for in a professional manner. They may engender feelings of anger, rejection, frustration, fear, or resentment on the part of the nurse. Taking care of such patients requires specific skills.

SPECIFIC SITUATIONS

1. **The Seductive Patient**
   Nurse response: At first naïveté, then confusion and embarrassment.
   Management tips:
   - Always have another person present, especially for genital exams.
   - Be wary of accepting gifts.
   - Be suspicious of frequent phone calls.
   - Terminate relationship if necessary. Have another nurse take over primary care.

2. **The Chronic Somatizer**
   Nurse response: Initially impatience, later rejection.
   Management tips:
   - Be alert to new symptoms.
   - Avoid unnecessary diagnostic procedures.
   - Minimize medication use.
   - A psychiatrist, psychologist, or advanced practice nurse (APN) may be an appropriate referral.

3. **The Manipulating Drug Abuser**
   Nurse response: Anger, resentment, frustration.
   Management tips:
   - Set limits and stick to them.
   - Be suspicious of strange stories about lost pills.
   - Refer to pain clinic or detoxification program if patient is willing.

4. **The Overly Dependent Patient**
   Nurse response: Gratification at first, then resentment.
   Management tips:
   - Be wary of the patient with extreme gratitude.

- Set firm limits for frequency of calls.
- Freely acknowledge to the patient your own human limitations.
- Set boundaries.

5. **The Terminally Ill Patient**

Nurse response: Impotence and frustration.

Management tips:

- Realize that the patient is looking for care, not cure.
- Ensure that adequate comfort care measures are maintained.
- Make an effort to be there for the patient and family.

6. **The Noncompliant or Nonadherent Patient**

Nurse response: Loss of control, then loss of interest.

Management tips:

- Recognize limitations in changing patient's behavior.
- Let go of your need to control.
- Resist the desire to give up.
- Change therapeutic plan to modalities that the patient will accept, realizing that the healthcare team may have to settle for less than optimal treatment.

7. **The Borderline Personality**

Nurse response: Anger and hostility.

Management tips:

- Refer for psychiatric co-care, but be aware of "splitting."
- Avoid drugs that are addictive.
- Set firm, but fair, limits and be consistent.

8. **The Abusive (Physically or Mentally) Personality**

Nurse response: Fear, anger and hostility.

Management tips:

- Refer for psychiatric co-care.
- If necessary, ask additional staff to be present when providing care.
- Notify patient's family and/or significant others.
- Request intervention from security staff, if necessary.

- Consult with institutional risk management, if necessary.
- Seek ethics consultation, if necessary.

SKILLS AND TECHNIQUES NEEDED TO MANAGE DIFFICULT PATIENTS

Those who are adept at managing difficult patients point out that when healthcare providers acknowledge their feelings toward these patients, they are better able to manage the patient's care. Recommendations include:

1. Stop denying intense or hateful feelings toward a patient.
2. Recognize countertransference.
3. Recognize that these feelings are, in a sense, part of the "diagnosis" for that particular patient.
4. Discuss feelings with colleagues in order to obtain their help.
5. Remember that, ultimately, it is not these feelings but how the nurse behaves toward the patient that is most important.

REFERENCES

Barsky AJ. Hidden reasons some patients visit doctors. *Ann Intern Med*. 1981;94:492-498.

Drossman DA. The problem patient. *Ann Intern Med*. 1978;88:366-372.

Groves JE. Taking care of the hateful patient. *N Engl J Med*. 1978;298:883-887.

Zollo MB, Derse AR. The abusive patient: where do you draw the line? *Am J Nurs*. 1997;97:31-35.

XIII. PAIN MANAGEMENT/PALLIATIVE CARE

ETHICAL ASPECTS OF NURSING CARE

Pain management in nursing practice revolves around issues of competence. Nurses must be able to competently assess and treat patients' pain. To do this, nurses must be cognizant of age-specific differences in pain management, as well as the patient's cultural response to pain. Nurses must have knowledge relevant to the current scope of nursing practice, changing issues and concerns, and ethical concepts and principles.

The individual nurse's knowledge and experience must be appropriate for his or her assigned responsibilities. It is important not only to develop competence as related to tasks and skills, but also to develop critical thinking and decision-making competence.

Additionally, nurses must recognize that the perception and expression of pain differ among cultures as well as among individual patients. Pain is more than a physiologic experience; it may have psychological and sociological dimensions as well. Nurses must consider culturally relevant aspects of pain within the patient population that they care for. It is important to see patients as individuals, not as a cultural group or as a representative of a cultural group.

THE NEED FOR MORE AGGRESSIVE TREATMENT

Many patients and family members fear that pain control may be inadequate (with good reason). The prevalence of this fear may be responsible, in part, for the increasing interest in euthanasia and assisted suicide.

MISTAKES THAT ARE MADE

1. The drug selection may be poor. For example, meperidine (Demerol) is clearly inferior to morphine for the control of the severe pain of bony metastases.
2. The dose may be inadequate or the dosing interval too long. For example, 75 milligrams of Demerol every 4 hours for postoperative pain in a 210-pound man is insufficient.
3. Physicians and nurses may fear causing addiction in patients with

chronic pain or terminal illness who must take large doses for long periods of time.

4. Physicians may prescribe inadequate doses of narcotics to patients who are terminally ill, for fear of inducing respiratory depression.

GOOD PAIN MANAGEMENT

1. **Choice/Dose of Drugs**

   Learn the appropriate drugs for given clinical situations and the proper dose and dosing interval.

2. **Knowledge about Addiction**

   Addiction (true psychological dependence) is rare in patients who receive narcotics for pain, even if the drug must be continued for protracted periods. Tolerance—the need to increase the dose for the same pharmacologic effect—varies from patient to patient. Physiologic dependence occurs in all patients with long-term use, but opioids can be tapered over several days to avoid withdrawal symptoms.

3. **Respiratory Depression**

   Hospices and oncology services report that respiratory depression is uncommon in patients who are receiving opioids for the control of pain; if present, it is often from some cause other than the opioid. Pain itself is a respiratory stimulant, and the opioid's effect on the respiratory center diminishes rapidly with chronic use. If the patient is terminally ill and the dose of opioid required to produce comfort does happen to depress respiration, it is still reasonable to allow the undesired effect (respiratory depression) in order to achieve the desired effect (relief of suffering).

4. **Terminal Sedation**

   Sometimes physicians and nurses may have to resort to this procedure to relieve the suffering of a dying patient whose disease is incurable and whose symptoms are refractory (cannot be controlled despite aggressive efforts that do not compromise consciousness). Symptoms requiring deep sedation for relief include:

   • Dyspnea (most common cause)

   • Pain not controlled by opioid without distressing side-effects

- Agitated delirium, restlessness with myoclonus
- Unrelieved vomiting

PLACEBOS

The use of placebos necessarily involves deception, which automatically raises serious ethical concerns. Primary tenets of ethical nursing practice include truth-telling, fidelity, trust, and respectful care. Informed consent, which most often is absent in the use of placebos, is a necessary requirement for promoting the autonomy of patients.

Even though the use of placebos often is contemplated out of a desire to benefit patients, this practice may ultimately compromise the therapeutic relationship between patients and healthcare providers by eroding the required environment of trust. Patients in pain are already vulnerable, and nurses should be persistent in their efforts to avoid increasing this vulnerability through inadequate pain management or deceptive communication.

The position of the Oncology Nursing Society (ONS) is that placebos should not be used to achieve the following:

1. To assess or manage cancer pain
2. To determine if the pain is "real"
3. To diagnose psychological symptoms, such as anxiety associated with pain

RECOMMENDATIONS

Healthcare providers have an ethical obligation to work to ensure that their institution has policies that address the use of placebos and prohibit deceptive use for assessment or management of pain in patients with cancer. Institutions need to develop educational programs to inform professionals about pain management, including the inappropriate use of placebos for cancer pain. Ethics committees can be helpful in case discussions regarding the use of placebos. It is important to use a multidisciplinary team to address complex issues in cancer pain management.

FURTHER READING

Hennepin County, Minnesota, Medical Society Policy Statement

"The administration of large quantities of narcotic analgesics is not euthanasia when the purpose is to alleviate pain and suffering, not to shorten the life of the patient. There are sufficient ethical, moral and medical reasons to prescribe morphine and other pain relieving medications even at the risk of hastening the patient's death.

"The goal of treatment is to relieve patient suffering to the fullest extent possible. For dying patients there is no 'cap' dose; high doses may be required for the relief of pain and suffering."

From Wanzer et al.

"In the patient whose dying process is irreversible, the balance between minimizing pain and suffering and potentially hastening death should be struck clearly in favor of pain relief. Narcotics and other pain medications should be given in whatever dose and by whatever route is necessary for relief. It is morally correct to increase the dose of narcotics to whatever dose is needed, even though the medication may contribute to the depression of respiration or blood pressure, the dulling of consciousness or even death, providing the primary goal of the physician is to relieve suffering. The proper dose of pain medication is the dose that is sufficient to relieve pain and suffering, even to the point of unconsciousness."

REFERENCES

Bleich JD. The ethics of pain management. *Cancer Invest.* 1994;12:362-363.

Breitbart W, Holland J. Psychiatric aspects of cancer pain. In: Foley KM , Bonica JJ, Ventafridda V, eds. *Advances in Pain Research and Therapy: Second International Congress on Cancer Pain.* Vol 16. New York: Raven Press; 1990:399-412.

Buchan ML, Tolle SW. Pain relief for dying persons: dealing with physicians' fears and concerns. *J Clin Ethics.* 1995;6:53-61.

Cherny NL, Portenoy RK. Sedation in the management of refractory symptoms: guidelines for evaluation and treatment. *J Palliative Care.* 1994;10:31-38.

Elander G. Ethical conflicts in placebo treatment. *J Adv Nurs.* 1991;16:947-951.

Graves SA, Berman LS. Caring for the child in a general postanesthesia care unit. *Am J Anesthesiol.* 1996;23:176-181.

Kachoyeanos MK, Zollo MB. Ethics in pain management of infants and children. *American Journal of Maternal Child Nursing.* 1995;20:142-147.

Kleinman I, Brown P, Librach L. Placebo pain medication: ethical and practical considerations. *Arch Fam Med.* 1994;3:453-457.

Lee B, Wheeler T. Emergence and recovery from anesthesia for pediatric patients in the postanesthesia care unit. *Pediatr Ann.* 1997;8:461-469.

McCaffery M, Ferrell BR. Nurses' knowledge about cancer pain: a survey of five countries. *J Pain & Symptom Manage.* 1995;10:356-369.

McCaffery M, Thorpe DM. Differences in perception of pain and the development of adversarial relationships among health care providers. In: Hill CS, Fields W, eds. *Advances in Pain Research and Therapy: Drug Treatment of Cancer Pain in a Drug-Oriented Society.* Vol 11. New York: Raven Press; 1989:19-26.

McGrath, PJ, Unruh, AM. Psychological treatment of pain in children and adolescents. In: Schechter NL, Berde CB, Yaster M, eds. *Pain in Infants, Children, and Adolescents.* Baltimore: Williams & Wilkins; 1993:219-228.

Meihart NT, McCaffery M. *Pain: A Nursing Approach for Assessment and Analysis.* Norwalk, Conn.: Appleton-Century-Crofts; 1983.

Melzack R. The tragedy of needless pain. *Sci Am.* 1990;262:27-33.

Melzack R, Wall P. *The Challenge of Pain.* London: Penguin Books; 1998.

Miser AW. Management of pain associated with childhood cancer. In: Schechter NL, Berde CB, Yaster M, eds. *Pain in Infants, Children and Adolescents.* Baltimore: Williams & Wilkins; 1993:411-424.

Quill TE, Lo B, Brock DW. Palliative options of last resort. *JAMA.* 1997;278:2099-2104.

Raj PP. *Practical Management of Pain.* 2nd ed. St. Louis: Mosby-Year Book; 1982.

Rothman KJ. Michels KB. The continuing unethical use of placebo controls. *N Engl J Med.* 1984;331:394-398.

Rousseau P. Terminal sedation in the care of dying patients. *Arch Intern Med.* 1996;156:1785-1786.

Rushton CH. Placebo pain medication: ethical and legal issues. *Pediatr Nurs.* 1985;21:166-168.

Wall PD. The placebo and the placebo response. In: Wall PD, Melzac R, eds. *Textbook of Pain.* 3rd ed. Edinburgh: Churchill; 1994:1297-1308.

Wanzer SH, et al. The physician's responsibility toward hopelessly ill patients: a second look. *N Engl J Med.* 1989;320:844-849.

XIV. FUTILITY/UNREASONABLE PATIENT REQUESTS

NATURE OF REQUESTS

Sometimes patients make unreasonable requests: a computed tomography (CT) scan for a tension headache or an antibiotic for a viral infection. Ethical principles substantiate the nurse's refusal to accede to a patient's demands to provide interventions that have no potential benefit or scientific merit—that is, those that are futile.

FUTILITY

Futility is difficult to define, but the following definition seems reasonable: "Medical futility means any effort to provide a benefit to a patient that is highly likely to fail and whose rare exceptions cannot systematically be reproduced" (Schneiderman and Jecker, 1995, p. 11).

Many ethicists believe that a distinction must be made between an *effect* that is limited to some part of the patient's body and the *benefit* that the patient has the capacity to appreciate and that improves the patient as a whole. For example, a ventilator that is effective in sustaining respiration may not be considered a benefit by a patient whose death from metastatic malignancy is imminent. Nonsentient patients (such as patients in a persistent vegetative state) cannot personally experience any intervention as a benefit.

The term *futility* refers to a specific medical intervention applied to a specific patient at a particular time. The term does not refer to a general situation of treatment or to a patient personally.

REASONS FOR REQUESTS FOR FUTILE OR IRRATIONAL THERAPY

1. **Unrealistic Goals of the Patient and/or Family**

   Physicians may fail to discuss achievable goals with the patient in terms of the change that would most likely result from the specific intervention being considered.

2. **Guilt**

   Families may worry about betrayal of patient trust if they agree to withdrawal of treatment. They may also be compensating for past neglect or inattention.

3. **Confusion in Formulation of the Therapeutic Plan**

    This situation is most likely to occur in serious illness with a multiplicity of consultants (and no one apparently in charge).

4. **Mistrust of Physicians by the Patient or Family**

    Involvement of the primary care physician who knows the patient well may resolve this.

5. **Ethnic and Socioeconomic Differences**

    Poor and minority patients may worry that any curtailment of services is rationing. They may be concerned about undertreatment as a form of discrimination.

6. **Denial Mechanisms of the Patient or Family**

    The patient or family may refuse to come to terms with reliable information.

7. **Misunderstandings/Language Barriers**

    If an interpreter is necessary, he or she should be an objective observer, preferably with some medical training—not a family member.

8. **Religious Issues**

    Family is awaiting or is certain of a miraculous cure.

RIGHTS OF PATIENTS

1. **Negative Rights (The Right of Refusal)**

    These are strong rights, and include the right of a decisional patient to refuse any and all treatment. These rights are based on liberty and privacy. Physicians are obligated to respect such refusals.

2. **Positive Rights (The Right to Request a Specific Treatment)**

    These rights are weaker because they impose an obligation on others. Patients cannot demand treatment that is considered futile by the physician because this would obligate the physician to violate his/her professional integrity in order to provide the useless treatment.

GROUNDS FOR REFUSAL OF AN UNREASONABLE REQUEST

A doctor or nurse may refuse a patient's request for the following reasons:

1. The request is for something that is outside the scope of good nursing practice or medical care. Such a judgment is based on the lack of objective evidence for effectiveness of the requested intervention.
2. The request requires the nurse or doctor to act illegally.
3. The request requires the nurse or doctor to violate a personal and professional standard of responsible medical practice.
4. The requested treatment cannot be anticipated to produce any beneficial result for this patient.

ADDITIONAL CAVEATS
1. When the request is for treatment that has reasonable potential for both benefit and harm, the preference of the fully informed patient must take precedence.
2. Decisions should not be made solely on the basis of economic considerations.
3. When a nurse or physician decides not to comply with a patient's request, a second opinion should usually be offered.

ETHICAL CONCERNS
1. "The right of the patient to choose does not imply the right to demand care beyond appropriate options based on medical judgment and accepted standards of care, nor are physicians required to provide care in ways that in their personal judgment violate the principles of medical ethics" (*JAMA*. 1992;268:2282-2288).
2. "The well being principle circumscribes the range of alternatives offered to patients: informed consent does not mean that patients can insist upon anything they might want. Rather, it is a choice among medically accepted and available options, all of which are believed to have some possibility of promoting the patient's welfare" (President's Commission for the Study of Ethical Problems in Medicine and Biomedical and Behavioral Research. 1982:42-44).

LEGAL CONCERNS
The law does not outline the standards for clinicians to use in or-

der to decide when to refuse an unreasonable patient request. Rather, the law articulates general duties that arise from the nurse-patient relationship and its ethical framework. The courts, through the laws of professional negligence, enforce these duties, maintaining that failure to fulfill them may result in compensable harm to the patient. The nurse's primary legal duty is broad and nonspecific. She or he must possess and apply the knowledge and use the skill and care that is ordinarily used by reasonably well-qualified nurses in similar circumstances. This does not mean that the nurse must acquiesce to patients' demands that are unreasonable.

Many nurses and doctors unreasonably fear liability for not "doing everything," such as instituting every available technology if the patient requests it. The law rarely dictates the particulars of clinical practice and does not require that healthcare providers do everything requested by a patient, agent, or guardian.

DIFFERENCE BETWEEN FUTILITY AND RATIONING

As Loewy points out, there is a danger that "futility" may be used as an excuse for decisions made on the basis of economic considerations—a real danger in a medical system driven by market forces.

It is particularly important to distinguish *futility*—a concept applied to a given patient and implying no apparent therapeutic benefit in that specific situation regardless of cost—from *rationing*—a concept that applies not to the individual but to society at large. Rationing also differs from futility in that it may acknowledge therapeutic benefit but deny it to some or all members of society because of cost.

THE NURSE'S RESPONSE TO FUTILE SITUATIONS

It may be best to avoid the term *futility* in discussion with patients. One might instead use phrases such as "this won't help," or "this might even cause more problems." It is often better to approach discussions with patients in ways that will answer three questions:

1. What are the realistic goals of this particular patient in these particular circumstances?

2. Is the treatment being considered likely to achieve these goals without undue burden?

3. Is the planned intervention consistent with the provision of good patient care?

Many requests for futile interventions result from incomplete or inadequate information. By spending time in careful communication with the patient (or surrogate) about reasonable expectations, nurses and doctors may avoid later confrontations. Healthcare providers ought not to feel obliged to provide unreasonable or inappropriate care just because it is requested by a patient. The decision not to provide treatment is made not because the patient no longer has any value or because the healthcare providers lack respect for the family's wishes. It is done because the care or treatment intervention requested is not medically indicated for the patient's condition.

REFERENCES

Alpers A, Lo B. Avoiding family feuds: responding to surrogate demands for life-sustaining interventions. *J Law, Med & Ethics*. 1999;27(1):74-80.

American Medical Association, Council on Ethical and Judicial Affairs. Guidelines for CPR: ethical considerations in resuscitation. *JAMA*. 1992;268:2282-2288.

Loewy EH, Carlson RA. Futility and its wider implications. *Arch Intern Med*. 1993;153:429-431.

Paris JJ. Pipes, colanders, and leaky buckets: reflections on the futility debate. *Cambridge Q Healthcare Ethics*. 1993;2:147-149.

President's Commission for the Study of Ethical Problems in Medicine and Biomedical and Behavioral Research. *Making Health Care Decisions: The Ethical and Legal Implications of Informed Consent in the Patient-Physician Relationship*. Washington, DC: US Government Printing Office; 1982:42-44.

Ruddick R. Hope and deception. *Bioethics*. 1999;13(3-4):343-357.

Schneiderman LJ, Jecker NS. Is the treatment beneficial, experimental or futile? *Cambridge Q Healthcare Ethics*. 1996;5:248-256.

Schneiderman LJ, Jecker NS. *Wrong Medicine*. Baltimore: Johns Hopkins University Press; 1995.

Schroeter K. Medical futility: Interpretation and ethical ramifications for the perioperative nurse. *Semin Perioperative Nurs*. 1997;6:138-141.

Shotton L. Can nurses contribute to better end-of-life care? *Nurs. Ethics*. 2000;7(2):134-140.

Wear S, Logue G. The problem of medically futile treatment: falling back on a preventive ethics approach. *J Clin Ethics*. 1995;6:138-148.

XV. ORGAN DONATION

NURSES' ROLE

It is a federal regulation that all patient deaths (including newborns who require a death certificate) be referred to an organ procurement organization (OPO) at the time of death or when imminent death has been established.

Many potential organ donors are victims of accidents and violent crimes that result in intracranial injury. Patients pronounced brain dead from subarachnoid hemorrhage, cerebrovascular accidents, primary brain tumor without metastasis, anoxic brain injury, drug overdose, smoke inhalation, drowning, or cardiac arrest should be considered potential donors. Because almost every potential organ donor is admitted to a hospital (or, in most cases, an intensive care unit), the nurse plays a central role in the donation process.

The role of the nurse is twofold:

1. Timely identification of potential donors
2. Referral of potential donors to the appropriate OPO

Through interactions with potential donors and their families, the nurse can serve as a bridge that provides a second chance at life to some of the thousands of individuals on the national organ transplant waiting list. While organ and bone marrow transplants can save lives, bone, cornea, heart valve, skin and other tissue transplants can improve the quality of life for many patients.

Although people often associate organ and tissue donation with the tragic loss of a loved one, many donors and their families view the decision to donate as a final and gratifying decision that will allow a patient to see for the first time, rescue a child from dialysis and allow her to play freely, or save a dying person's life.

Additionally, nurses must be sensitive to and honor the requests of persons who do not desire to donate because of their personal or cultural beliefs.

SUITABLE DONORS

1. In most states, anyone over the age of 18 can become a donor simply by signing a donor card. Some states require witnesses to this signature.
2. Organs may be donated from someone as young as a newborn.

However, those under 18 can become donors only with parental permission. (This is true even if the donor is 16 and has signed the donor card section on his or her driver's license.)

3. A person is never considered too old to be a donor. In the past there were age restrictions, but now the only true limit to donation is the condition of the organs. However, normal tissue protocols typically limit donation to the age of 70.

TRANSPLANTABLE ORGANS
1. Kidney
2. Liver
3. Heart
4. Lung
5. Pancreas
6. Small bowel

TRANSPLANTABLE TISSUES
1. Skin
2. Bone
3. Heart valves
4. Veins
5. Fascia
6. Cornea
7. Bone marrow

CRITERIA FOR ORGAN DONATION
1. Solid organ donors must meet the criteria for brain death and must be on ventilator support.
2. The issue of non-heart-beating donors (NHBDs) remains controversial but is current policy at some institutions. In these patients, the ventilator is discontinued; hypotension, apnea, and cardiac standstill ensue; and the patient is pronounced dead by heart-lung death criteria. Organ recovery begins directly after this process. This protocol is often seen to blur some of the clear lines established by brain death protocols—thus the controversy.

3. Bone and tissue donation occurs within 24 hours of death.
4. Eye donation ideally occurs within 4 to 6 hours of death.
5. Patients with infection, sepsis, or an active malignancy are not candidates for organ donation.
6. These criteria are quite flexible. Organs and tissues from older donors are used more now than in the past.

CONSENT FOR ORGAN DONATION

1. Legally, a signed donor card takes precedence over the wishes of any survivor. The donor's wishes should be explained to the family.
2. The family of any potential donor (who does not have a specific contraindication to donation) must be asked about donation and should be encouraged to give permission (especially when the patient is brain dead and is thus a suitable donor for solid organs).
3. Even if the person did not sign the driver's license for organ donation, the family may agree to donate organs.

COST OF ORGAN DONATION

Families need to be told that they are not responsible for any of the costs related to the donation process.

FUNERAL ARRANGEMENTS AFTER ORGAN DONATION

1. Assure the family that the body is released soon after the organs and/or tissues are recovered and that funeral arrangements are rarely delayed.
2. When donation is complete, prosthetic replacements are used to restore the body to its natural appearance. Open-casket viewing is possible with any type of donation.

INSTITUTIONAL RESOURCES

All institutions have access to someone with expertise in organ and tissue donation who can give advice. A phone call to the OPO on call is recommended before approaching the next of kin regarding donation.

FURTHER READING

Organ Commerce

Another ethical issue in transplantation is the buying and selling of human organs. The National Organ Transplant Act of 1984 prohibits the purchase or sale of human organs and tissues. In addition, the Uniform Anatomical Gift Act (UAGA) of each state forbids the sale or purchase of parts or organs. The idea that it is permissible to sell some body parts (such as sperm and blood plasma) and not others is highlighted in these debates. The critics of commerce in organ transplantation postulate that exploitation, coercion, and violations of the sanctity of the person as a human being would occur with such a practice.

Prisoners as Organ Donors or Recipients

The critical shortage of organs for transplantation continues to force the medical community to explore atypical solutions that raise a number of ethical concerns. It has been suggested, even proposed in the form of legislation, that prisoners (particularly death-row inmates) be allowed to donate organs. This volatile discussion is not restricted to developing nations. In the United States it has been suggested that condemned prisoners be allowed to trade an organ for a reduction in sentence (from death to life in prison). Ethical issues include informed consent of potential donors and recipients, prisoners' ability to make a coercion-free decision, discrimination against individuals found to be medically unsuitable, and the effect of such policies on our current altruistic donation practices.

Allocation Concerns

Once an individual is evaluated and accepted as a candidate for transplant, the wait for a donated organ begins. As donated organs become available, they are allocated in a prescribed manner set forth in United Network for Organ Sharing (UNOS) Organ Procurement and Transplantation policies. The UNOS organ allocation system is based on the ethical principles of justice (equity) and medical utility and strives to balance these principles.

The UAGA of each state delineates who may give and who may receive donated organs. Yet there is some variation in the ability of individuals to direct a donation. The UNOS Board of Directors approved a recommendation made by its ethics committee in June 1996 dealing with the subject of directed donation. The committee recommended for incorporation to the Commissioners for Uniform Acts the following statement: "Donation of an organ may not be made in a manner which discriminates against a person or class of persons on the basis of race, national origin, religion, gender or similar characteristic."

Consent Issues

The UAGA outlines a consent process for donation. It describes who can complete this process and provides a vehicle—the donor card—for the process. The donor card, by virtue of the UAGA, is a legal document. Nonetheless, OPOs in the United States rarely act solely on the presence of a donor card. The majority of organ recovery agencies seek permission from the next of kin for donation, even when the potential donor has signed a donor card.

Non-Heart-Beating Donors (NHBDs)

Another category of organ donors consists of patients who have suffered circulatory and respiratory death. This concept isn't novel and is the basis on which modern clinical transplantation was formed. It has been nearly 20 years since this type of organ donor has been utilized. These potential organ donors are classified as NHBDs because the beating of the heart has ceased at the time of organ recovery. NHBDs generally fall into two categories: controlled and uncontrolled. *Controlled* NHBDs are maintained on artificial ventilation or, on some occasions, circulatory assistance. These patients suffer irreversible cessation of circulatory and respiratory functions within a short interval after withdrawal of support. *Uncontrolled* NHBDs include patients who have experienced a cardiorespiratory arrest outside or within the hospital and cannot be resuscitated, and patients who are presumed to be brain dead who arrest prior to completion of brain death criteria or arrest after brain death has been declared, but prior to the recovery of organs.

REFERENCES

American Medical Association, Council on Ethical and Judicial Affairs. Ethical considerations in the allocation of organs and other scarce medical resources among patients. *Arch Intern Med.* 1995; 155: 29-40.

Bernat JL. *Resolving Ethical Dilemmas: A Guide for Clinicians.* Baltimore, Md: Williams & Wilkins; 1995.

Cranford RE. Brain death. In: Phillips MG, ed. *Organ Procurement, Preservation and Distribution in Transplantation.* Richmond, Va: The William Byrd Press, Inc.; 1991: 23-31.

Cohen C, Benjamin M. Alcoholics and liver transplantation. *JAMA.* 1991; 265: 1299-1301.

Dennis JM, Hanson P, Hodge EE, Krom RAF, Veatch RM. An evaluation of the ethics of presumed consent and a proposal based on required response. *UNOS Update.*1994; 10: 16-21.

Institute of Medicine. *Non-Heart-Beating Organ Donation: Medical and Ethical Issues in Procurement.* Washington, DC: National Academy Press; 1997.

Lo B. *Resolving Ethical Dilemmas: A Guide for Clinicians.* Baltimore, Md: Williams & Wilkins; 1995.

Lu L. Commerce in organ transplantation. *The Pharos.* 1998; 61: 2-5.

Moss AH, Siegler M. Should alcoholics compete equally for liver transplantation? *JAMA.* 1991; 265:1295-1298.

Schroeter K, Taylor G. Ethical considerations for the critical care nurse. *Critical Care Nurse.*1999;2:60-69.

Taylor GJ. Organs for all. *Hasting Cent Rep.* 1997; 27: 46-47.

Ubel PA, Arnold RA, Caplan AL. Rationing failure: the ethical lessons of retransplantation of scarce vital organs. *JAMA.* 1993; 270: 2469-2474.

Wilkinson S, Garrad E. Bodily integrity and the sale of human organs. *J Med Ethics.*1995; 22: 334-9.

Youngner SJ, Arnold RM. Ethical, psychological, and public policy implications of procuring organs from non-heart beating cadaver donors. *JAMA.* 1993; 269: 2769-2774.

XVI. ADVANCE DIRECTIVES

DEFINITION

An advance directive (AD) is a statement a patient makes, while still in possession of decision-making capacity, about how treatment decisions should be made at some future time if he or she loses the capacity to make such decisions.

TYPES OF ADs

1. Living will (LW) statutory form
2. Power of attorney for healthcare (PAHC) statutory form
3. Nonstatutory forms

LIVING WILL

1. **Provisions**

   Most statutory forms are documents stating the desire to die a "natural" death and not to be kept alive by medical treatment and machines. In many states, the principal may also stipulate that fluids and nutrition are to be discontinued in the event of persistent vegetative state (PVS).

2. **Activation**

   Usually the LW becomes effective on the determination of "terminal" illness or "imminent" death or the diagnosis of PVS made by two physicians.

POWER OF ATTORNEY FOR HEALTHCARE

1. **Provisions**

   Most statutory forms provide a way for the principal to appoint a person to act as healthcare agent, proxy, or surrogate to make healthcare decisions in the event that the principal loses the capacity to make decisions. The PAHC allows the principal to add specific directions, and often the agent may be given authority to have feeding tubes withheld or withdrawn (even in the absence of PVS).

2. **Activation**

   The PAHC becomes effective when two physicians, or (in most jurisdictions) one physician and one psychologist, determine that the principal is no longer decisional.

PREFERENCE

Patients may ask for the physician's advice about ADs. The statutory form of the PAHC is the best choice because it allows all of the options of a LW and has the added advantage of providing an agent— someone who knows the principal well and can take an active role in the decision-making process on the patient's behalf. The PAHC also allows for the addition of specific instructions to the agent. There is no advantage to filling out both forms. The forms require the signatures of adult witnesses (usually two).

Depending on the type of form used, AD forms do not always require a fee for processing. Forms are available at no cost from various sources such as hospitals (usually social services departments), clergy or religious organizations, Internet sites, and legal offices.

Note: The laws regarding LWs and PAHCs vary from state to state. Nurses should check the provisions and standards for activation in their own jurisdictions.

FURTHER READING

Living Will
  Strengths
  - Allows the physician to understand the patient's wishes and motivations.
  - Extends the patient's autonomy, self-control, and self-determination.
  - Relieves the patient's anxiety about unwanted treatment.
  - Provides legal immunity for physicians who follow dictates in good faith.
  - Reduces family strife and sense of guilt.
  - Improves communication and trust between patient and physician.

  Weaknesses
  - Applicable only to those in PVS or the terminally ill (patients who have a disease that is incurable and will die regardless of treatment).
  - Death must be imminent (likely to occur within 6 months).
  - Ambiguous terms may be difficult to interpret later.
  - There is no proxy decision maker, so:
    - It requires prediction of final illness scenario and available treatment.
    - It requires physician to make decisions on the basis of an interpretation of a document.

Power of Attorney for Healthcare (PAHC)
  1. Activation of PAHC

Lack of decision-making capacity must be certified by two physicians or (in most jurisdictions) one physician and a psychologist who have examined the patient. Until then, the patient makes all the decisions.

2. **Advantages**
   - Physician has someone to talk with—a proxy, a knowledgeable surrogate—who can provide a substituted judgment of how the patient would have chosen. If the agent is unable to provide a substituted judgment, the agent and physician together can use the best-interest standard (how a reasonable person might choose in consideration of the benefit-burden concept of proportionality).
   - Provides flexibility; this decreases ambiguity and uncertainty because there is no way to predict all possible scenarios.
   - Authority of agent can be limited as person desires.
   - Avoids family conflict about rightful agent.
   - Provides legal immunity for physicians who follow dictates in good faith.
   - Allows appointment of a nonrelative (especially valuable for persons who may be alienated from their families).
   - Most forms can be completed without an attorney.

Nonstatutory Forms

These are forms that are not codified in state law. They may contain ambiguous language, which can cause difficulty in interpretation. In many states, nonstatutory forms—unlike the statutory forms of the LW and PAHC—may not provide legal immunity for physicians who follow the dictates of the document.

Patient Self-Determination Act (PSDA)

This federal law, which went into effect in 1991, involves all Medicare and Medicaid providers (hospitals, nursing homes, hospices, and health-maintenance organizations).

According to the provisions of the PSDA, all healthcare providers must:
1. Give all patients written information at the time of admission, advising them of their rights to refuse any treatments and to have an AD. This is usually done by nursing or social service staff shortly after admission, but patients may ask physicians about ADs.
2. Document the presence of an AD in the patient's record.
3. Have written policies respecting the rights of patients to have an AD and to refuse treatment.
4. Make provisions to educate staff and community regarding these issues.
5. Prohibit discrimination against individuals because they do or do not have an AD.

Some Misconceptions Patients Have about ADs

1. "If I sign one, I can't change my mind."

   An AD can easily be revoked—orally, in writing, or by filling out a new AD that supersedes the old.

2. "I'm young and/or I'm in good health, so I don't need an AD."

    The *Cruzan* and *Quinlan* cases—two prominent court cases that drew attention of the public to this issue—involved women in their 20s.

3. "If I have an AD, paramedics would not resuscitate me."

    Because the standard of activation for the LW is the presence of a terminal condition and for the PAHC is loss of decision-making capacity, these documents, as a rule, do not speak to emergency situations; insufficient time exists to determine the presence of the effective activating elements. An occasional exception is the chronically ill individual who specifies do-not-resuscitate in the PAHC.

4. "My family might not want me to sign an AD."

    Families generally welcome the opportunity to discuss these issues, and the presence of an AD can do much to relieve family guilt if it becomes necessary to withdraw or withhold treatment.

5. "My spouse/family knows what I want" or "My physician knows what I want."

    Numerous surveys report that neither family members nor physicians are accurate in their estimation of patients' preferences. Designation of an agent with specific instructions is the best way to circumvent this problem.

6. "The provisions of the AD may require me and/or my healthcare providers to act counter to my philosophy and conscience."

    The healthcare team members need to discuss the AD with the patient to make sure that no conflict exists between the patient's desires and the team members' principles. If a conflict is present, it may be necessary to transfer the patient to the care of another physician or team.

7. "I haven't had time to go to a lawyer to complete the forms."

    Many people believe that they must have these forms completed by lawyers. However, in many states, the forms can be completed without the assistance of others, or with the assistance of clergy or social workers.

Recommendations to Patients and the Public Regarding ADs

1. Think about the issues and your specific wishes. Discuss them with family.
2. Complete the PAHC form rather than the LW form.
3. Discuss your desires fully with both the primary and alternate agents. You may want to add some written instructions.
4. Discuss the decisions with your personal physician to get agreement on specifics.
5. Circulate these documents widely. Copies of the document should be given to primary and alternate agents, close family members, personal physician, and personal attorney.
6. Specific instructions can be added, such as the following example:

    "I value a full life more than a long life. If I have lost the ability to interact with others and have no reasonable chance of regaining this ability; or if my suffering is intense and irreversible, even though I have no terminal illness, I do not want to have my life prolonged. I would not then ask to be subjected to surgery or to resuscitation procedures, to intensive care services, or to other life-prolonging measures, including the administration of antibiotics, blood products or artificial nutrition and hydration" (Bok).

Nursing Implications

1. The healthcare institution is required by federal law to ask patients at the time of admission if they have ADs. The healthcare institution may delegate this duty to nurses. Although this is not always the most opportune time (obviously it may be better to discuss the issue of an AD at a more nonthreatening time), the first steps in obtaining an AD may begin at this point. The nurse may refer the patient to the physician, social services, or chaplaincy for assistance. Use of printed informational material is helpful, as is the availability of PAHC forms in the institution.
2. The nurse may describe the settings or situations in which an AD is important. The nurse may also tell patients that their physician will be in a better position to direct their treatment with a written AD.
3. Assure patients that symptomatic care and treatment will never be withheld.
4. Patients may need time to reflect and discuss these issues with their families. It may be a good idea to tell them that they can think about completing the AD so they do not feel as if they are rushing through it.
5. Document a patient's oral statements if an AD is not completed. If an AD is completed, file it in the patient's record.
6. Review the AD with the patient or surrogate to prevent misunderstandings.
7. Emphasize the need for the patient to discuss the AD fully with his or her family.
8. Complete an AD (PAHC) yourself.

REFERENCES

Bok S. Personal directions for care at the end of life. *N Engl J Med.* 1976;295:362-369.

Caralis PV, et al. The influence of ethnicity and race on attitudes toward advance directives, life-prolonging treatments, and euthanasia. *J Clin Ethics.* 1993;4:155-165.

Emanuel LL, et al. Advance directives for medical care: a case for greater use. *N Engl J Med.* 1991;324:889-895.

Gillich MR, et al. Medical technology at the end of life: what would physicians and nurses want for themselves? *Arch Intern Med.* 1993;153:2542-2547.

Lo B. Improving care near the end of life: why is it so hard? *JAMA.* 1995;274:1634-1636.

Lynn J, et al. Perceptions by family members of the dying experience of older and seriously ill patients. *Ann Intern Med.* 1997;126:97-106.

Miles SH, Koepp R, Weber EP. Advance end-of-life treatment planning. *Arch Intern Med.* 1996;156:1062-1068.

Pearlman RA, et al. Insights pertaining to patient assessments of states worse than death. *J Clin Ethics.* 1993;4:33-41.

Pearlman RA, Uhlmann RF, Jecker NS. Spousal understanding of patient quality of life: implications for surrogate decisions. *J Clin Ethics.* 1992;3:114-120.

XVII. AIDS

Ethical dilemmas encountered in the care of patients with acquired immunodeficiency syndrome (AIDS) may include issues of compassion, medical futility, care of the incompetent patient, confidentiality, and management of the difficult patient.

NURSES' RESPONSE TO THE AIDS RISK

Health professionals' fear of contracting AIDS will exist as long as there is a risk that the human immunodeficiency virus (HIV) can be transmitted in the healthcare setting. Despite infection control procedures, a very small (much less than 1%) occupational risk exists. This risk requires a professional response: nurses have always had to set aside personal fears in order to take care of sick persons.

The nurse may also have to overcome personal antipathies to patients of different cultural and socioeconomic background (such as intravenous drug users) and different sexual orientations. If a gap exists between nurse and patient, ethical discussions regarding the patient's preferences, allocation of resources, and use of cardiopulmonary resuscitation (CPR) are made more difficult.

The American Medical Association Council on Ethical and Judicial Affairs has stated, "A physician may not ethically refuse to treat a patient whose condition is within the physician's current realm of competence solely because the patient is seropositive. Persons who are seropositive should not be subjected to discrimination based on fear or prejudice" (*JAMA*. 1988;259:1360-1361). Federal laws contain similar conditions.

RECOMMENDATIONS FOR NURSES

1. Most patients with HIV infection benefit from combined drug therapy, which requires highly specialized clinical knowledge. For this reason, most HIV-positive patients are followed by infectious disease specialists. Nurses should learn as much about the disease as possible.

2. In many cases, nurses must try to bridge the social or psychological gap between themselves and their patients.

3. New treatment regimens have decreased the morbidity and mor-

tality of HIV infection, and AIDS is now becoming more of a chronic rather than a terminal disease.

4. Sometimes, however, treatment becomes futile. A decision should then be made to withdraw or withhold the treatment, using the skills and paradigms described in this text. Encouraging the patient to complete an advance directive helps decision making in these circumstances.

THE NURSE'S RESPONSIBILITIES TO PATIENTS WITH AIDS

1. Provide competent nursing care.
2. Safeguard patients and avoid actions that place the interests of patients in jeopardy.

The right to refuse an assignment should be narrowly construed, and the nurse must balance such a refusal against the obligation to provide for patients' safety and to avoid abandonment. A refusal of an assignment may be justified only when the risk of harm to the patient is greater by accepting the assignment than by rejecting it.

Health problems such as hepatitis B or C, tuberculosis, HIV/AIDS, cytomegalovirus, and other infectious processes may present the nurse with questions regarding when personal risk outweighs responsibility for care of the patient. The general principle of practice is that nurses are morally obligated to care for all patients. However, in certain cases the risks of harm may outweigh a nurse's responsibility to care for a given patient. In ethics, the differentiation between benefiting another as a moral duty and benefiting another as a moral option is found in four fundamental criteria.

As applied to nursing, a moral obligation exists for the nurse if all four of the following criteria are present:

- The patient is at significant risk of harm, loss, or damage if the nurse does not assist.
- The nurse's intervention or care is directly relevant to preventing harm.
- The nurse's care will probably prevent harm, loss, or damage to the patient.

• The benefit the patient will gain outweighs any harm the nurse might incur and does not present more than an acceptable risk to the nurse.

REFERENCES

American Medical Association, Council on Ethical and Judicial Affairs. Ethical issues involved in the growing AIDS crisis. *JAMA.* 1988;259:1360-1361.

American Nurses Association. *Code of Ethics for Nurses with Interpretive Statements.* Kansas City, Mo: ANA; 2001.

American Nurses Association. *Guidelines on reporting incompetent, unethical or illegal practices.* Washington, DC: ANA; 1994.

American Nurses Association. Standards of clinical nursing practice. Kansas City, Mo: ANA; 1991.

Callahan JC, Powell J. Nursing and AIDS: some special challenges. Cohen ED, Davis M, eds. *AIDS: Crisis in Professional Ethics.* Philadelphia: Temple University Press; 1994:51-73.

Daniels N. HIV-infected professionals, patient rights, and the switching dilemma. *JAMA.*1992; 267:1386-1371.

Derse AR. HIV and AIDS: legal and ethical issues in the emergency department. *Emerg Med Clin North Am.* 1995;13:213-223.

Freedman B. Violating confidentiality to warn of a risk of HIV infection: ethical work in progress. *Theoretical Medicine.* 1991; 12(4): 309-23.

Gorlin RA, ed. *Codes of Professional Responsibility.* 2nd ed., Washington, DC: Georgetown University Press; 1990.

Haas JS, et al. Discussions of preferences for life-sustaining care by persons with AIDS. *Arch Intern Med.* 1993;153:1241-1248.

Loeb S, et al. Nurse's handbook of law and ethics. Springhouse, Pa: Springhouse Corp; 1992.

McCloskey J, Grace H. *Current Issues in Nursing.* 4th ed. St. Louis, Mo: Mosby Publications; 1994.

Slim J. AIDS, nursing and occupational risk: an ethical analysis. *J Adv Nurs.* 1992;17:569-575.

Steinbrook R, et al. Ethical dilemmas in caring for patient with the acquired immunodeficiency syndrome. *Ann Intern Med.* 1985;103:787-790.

Wachter RM, Luce JM, Hopewell PC. Critical care of patients with AIDS. *JAMA.* 1992;267:541-547.

Wilson R, Crouch E. *Risk/Benefit Analysis.* Cambridge, Mass: Ballinger Publishing; 1982.

Zuger A, Miles SH. Physicians, AIDS, and occupational risk: historic traditions and ethical obligations. *JAMA.* 1987;258:1924-1928.

XVIII. DEATH CRITERIA

HEART-LUNG DEATH

The centuries-old determination of death is the heart-lung standard. All 50 states recognize heart-lung death—the cessation of heartbeat and respirations—as death.

STEPS IN PRONOUNCING DEATH

When a physician is called to pronounce a patient dead, the following steps are usually observed:

1. Code status is ascertained.
2. The patient is assessed for hypothermia or drug overdose, which can be confounding factors.
3. Auscultation for respirations and heart tones is performed.
4. Corneal reflexes are assessed with a wisp of cotton or tissue.
5. The patient is pronounced dead if no positive responses are found to any of the above. The time of death must be documented in the chart.

BRAIN DEATH

By definition, "whole brain" death occurs when the entire brain—including the cerebral cortex and the brain stem—has died. This definition of death has been endorsed by the American Medical Association and the American Bar Association.

IMPLICATIONS FOR NURSES

One ever-present topic for ethical debate in the organ donation arena is brain death (see section XV, p. 62).

The Uniform Determination of Death Act, accepted in every state since 1985, states: "An individual is considered dead, if sustaining either:

1. Irreversible cessation of circulatory and respiratory function, or
2. Irreversible cessation of all functions of the entire brain, including the brain stem." [The irreversible cessation of the functions of the entire brain is a legally accepted standard for de-

termining death when the use of mechanical ventilation precludes using traditional cardiopulmonary criteria.]

A different set of criteria is recognized for diagnosing brain death in children and infants as young as 6 months of age. Following any declaration of death, medical treatment would normally be discontinued. Such termination of treatment would include any type of ventilatory support.

In the organ-donation process where there is a need to make preparations to carry out the wishes of the donor (or to allow decision makers to consider the option of donation) and to preserve the organs for transplantation, the potential donor is physiologically supported following the declaration of death. This practice sets the framework for further ethical deliberation regarding decision making, harms and benefits, and distribution of risks and costs.

CRITERIA FOR DIAGNOSIS
1. A neurologic event adequate to produce brain death
2. Reliable examination showing absence of brain-stem function

FINDINGS ON PHYSICAL EXAMINATION
1. Profound coma ("eyes-closed unconsciousness")
2. No eye movement; no pupillary response
3. No corneal reflexes
4. No cough or gag reflex; no motor response to pain
5. No spontaneous respiratory attempts off the ventilator (There are several ways of testing for apnea. If the patient is a potential organ donor, this test should only be done after consultation with the transplant coordinator.)

LABORATORY CONFIRMATION
1. Radionuclide tracer shows no cerebral blood flow.
2. Electroencephalogram (EEG) is not reliable, especially in cases of drug overdose or hypothermia.

LEGAL ASPECTS

If above criteria are satisfied, the patient is legally dead and no further treatment is necessary. It is important to document the time of death in the chart before turning off the ventilator.

HUMANITARIAN ASPECTS

Patients who are brain dead may not *look* dead. It is important to work with the family to help them acknowledge the death of their loved one. Occasionally, the ventilator needs to be left on for a short time to allow for this adjustment. If the patient is in the intensive care unit (ICU), it may be possible to transfer him or her to a more comfortable room on a nursing unit where the family will feel more at ease about gathering at the patient's bedside. Family members and friends sometimes feel that the ICU setting is "too cold" or that they will be "disturbing" others.

CONTROVERSIES

There is some controversy about whether patients with loss of cerebral cortical function but with a functioning brain stem should be included in an expanded definition of brain death (see also criteria of death in organ donation, section XV, p. 62). Whether one chooses to believe in a "whole or higher" form, the term *brain death* may well be responsible for some of the confusion in addressing what is actually a neurological determination of death. This controversy will continue until clinicians reach consensus on the language and principles defining brain death.

REFERENCES

Coyle MA. Meeting the needs of the family: the role of the specialist nurse in the management of brain death. *Intensive & Crit Care Nurs.* 2000;16(1):45-50.

Firsching R. Moral dilemmas of tetraplegia; the 'locked-in' syndrome, the persistent vegetative state and brain death. *Spinal Cord.* 1998;36:741-743.

Frid I, Bergbom-Engberg I, Haljamae H. Brain death in ICUs and associated nursing care challenges concerning patients and families. *Intensive & Crit Care Nurs.* 1998;14(1):21-29.

Halevy A, Brody B. Brain death: reconciling definitions, criteria, and tests. *Ann Intern Med.* 1993;119:519-525.

O'Reilly A. A day in the life. *Maryland Nurs.* 2000;3(2):36-37.

Recommendations for managing vital-organ donors. *Dimens Crit Care Nurs.* 1999;18(2):13-15.

Veatch RM. The impending collapse of the whole-brain definition of death. *Hastings Cent Rep.* 1993;23:18-24.

Vitacco J, et al. Clinical viewpoints: clinical care nurses share how they cope with caring for the brain-dead pregnant woman. *Dimens Crit Care Nurs.* 1994;13(3):135-136.

XIX. EUTHANASIA AND ASSISTED SUICIDE

DEFINITIONS

1. **Euthanasia**

   The physician, nurse, or advanced practice nurse (APN) participates in an intentional, deliberate act to cause the immediate death of a person with terminal, incurable, or painful disease by the medical administration of a lethal drug.

2. **Assisted Suicide**

   The physician, nurse, or APN provides the lethal drug with instructions for its use but is not the agent. The patient decides when and if to use the drug.

   Most, but not all, ethicists agree that euthanasia and assisted suicide differ from one another significantly because of the agency. In euthanasia, the physician is the direct agent; in assisted suicide, the patient is the direct agent.

LEGAL ASPECTS

Euthanasia is illegal in all states. Suicide is not illegal, but all states except Oregon now have some sort of legal prohibition against assisted suicide. In all other states there is a specific law against assisting a suicide or prosecution is possible under other existing statutes or common law.

ETHICAL ASPECTS

1. **American Medical Association Policy:**

   "The intentional termination of the life of one human being by another is contrary to public policy, medical tradition, and the most fundamental measures of human value and worth" (AMA, *Euthanasia*).

2. **American College of Physicians Ethics Manual:**

   "Although a patient may refuse a medical intervention and the physician may comply with this refusal, the physician must never intentionally and directly cause death or assist a patient to commit suicide" (*Ann Intern Med.* 1989;111:245-335).

STATE INITIATIVES

In 1994, Oregon passed a ballot measure to allow physician assistance in suicide for suffering patients with terminal illness. For several years, it was not implemented because of legal challenge. Oregon voters in 1997 reaffirmed support (60% to 40%), and the federal appeals court lifted the injunction. Thus, Oregon is the only state in which physician-assisted suicide (but not euthanasia) is legal.

In 1997, the US Supreme Court rendered unanimous decisions that the state statutes against assisted suicide did not violate either the "due process" or "equal protection" provisions of the 14th Amendment of the US Constitution. The opinions of several Supreme Court justices affirmed the following:

1. Competent patients have the right to discontinue or to withhold any treatment, even that considered life sustaining.
2. Competent patients have the right to receive sufficient medication to relieve pain, even if that treatment causes shortening of the patient's life.
3. Competent patients whose suffering cannot otherwise be relieved have the right to have terminal sedation.
4. Because none of the above actions are considered suicide, physicians who accede to such patient requests cannot be considered to be "assisting a suicide."

The Court also allowed that the issue is not settled and that individual state legislatures might take future action legitimizing assisted suicide. Further attempts will undoubtedly follow. Because this issue will not go away, physicians, nurses, and other healthcare providers need to consider thoughtfully the professional response to this situation.

ETHICAL DISCUSSION

It is the responsibility of caring nurses and physicians to analyze the stimuli for these initiatives that have such public support and to attempt to change factors that are amenable to change. Prominent public fears that fuel this debate include the following:

1. The concern that the pain experienced by a terminally ill patient will not be controlled adequately

2. The worry about loss of control and the indignity of depen-
    dence during the final phase of the illness
3. The concern that medical technology will continue to be used
    inappropriately, thus delaying an "easy" death.

By providing adequate pain control to terminally ill patients without fearing addiction or respiratory depression, physicians will help as-
suage the first concern. Use of appropriate palliative measures and increased reliance on hospice care will relieve the other concerns. By
strongly recommending the use of advance directives and discussing
these issues with their patients, clinicians can reduce the burden of end-
of-life decision making.

If all of these interventions are carried out successfully, the stimu-
lus for state initiatives should decrease. However, regardless of the effectiveness of good pain control and palliative care, there will remain a
small but significant group of patients for whom no alternative to death
is acceptable and for whom aid in dying may not be considered, by
some, to be irrational. Each physician and nurse will have to decide
what the appropriate response will be.

NURSING FOCUS

The American Nurses Association (ANA) *Code for Nurses* states
that the nurse has a moral obligation to prevent and relieve the suffering
of dying patients but must never act deliberately to terminate the life of
any person. Nurses have a central role in assessing the presence of pain
in the dying patient and ensuring that the patient at the end of life has
pain controlled to an acceptable (from the patient's perspective) level.

The ANA's position statement, *Promotion of Comfort and Relief of
Pain in Dying Patients* (1991), directs nurses to use full and effective
doses of pain medication to achieve adequate symptom control, even if
death is hastened as a result. In this situation, relief of pain and promotion of comfort is the intended effect, and the hastening of death may
result secondarily from the drug's side-effects on consciousness and respiration. For the dying patient, the relief of pain and promotion of
comfort is a primary goal; administering increasing doses of medication
to achieve this goal is ethical, even when the risks of death are increased

(President's Commission for the Study of Ethical Problems in Medicine, 1983). Nurses understand the moral differences between the actions of providing effective pain relief to a dying patient and participating in euthanasia or assisted suicide.

REFERENCES

American College of Physicians. Ethics manual, part I: history, patient, other physicians. *Ann Intern Med.* 1989;111:245-335.

American Medical Association, Council on Ethical and Judicial Affairs. Decisions near the end of life. *JAMA.* 1992;267:2229-2233.

American Medical Association, Council on Ethical and Judicial Affairs. *Euthanasia.* Chicago: American Medical Association; June 1988. Report 12:1-40.

American Nurses Association. *Active Euthanasia* [position statement]. 1994. Available at <www.ana.org/readroom/position/ethics/eteuth.htm>.

American Nurses Association. *Assisted Suicide* [position statement].1994. Available at <www.ana.org/readroom/position/ethics/etsuic.htm>.

American Nurses Association. *Code for Nurses with Interpretive Statements.* Kansas City, Mo: ANA; 1985.

American Nurses Association. *Nursing's Social Policy Statement.* Washington, DC: ANA, 1995.

American Nurses Association. *Promotion of Comfort and Relief of Pain in the Dying Patient* [position statement]. 1991. Available at www.ana.org/readroom/position/ethics/etpain.htm>.

Brody H. Assisted death: a compassionate response to a medical failure. *N Engl J Med.* 1992;327:1384-1388.

Brody H. Causing, intending, and assisting death. *J Clin Ethics.* 1993;4:112-117.

Miller FC. A communitarian approach to physician assisted death. *Cambridge Q Healthcare Ethics.* 1997;6:78-87.

Nurse Avoids Prison in VA Overdoses. *Washington Post.* May 31, 2000:B2.

Orentlicher D. The legalization of physician assisted suicide. *JAMA.* 1996;335:663-667.

Quill TE, Cassel CK, Meier DE. Care of the hopelessly ill: proposed clinical criteria for physician assisted suicide. *N Engl J Med.* 1992;327:1380-1383.

Quill TE, Lo B, Brock DW. Palliative options of last resort: a comparison of voluntarily stopping eating and drinking, terminal sedation, physician-assisted suicide, and voluntary active euthanasia. *JAMA.* 1997;278:2099-2104.

President's Commission for the Study of Ethical Problems in Medicine and Biomedical and Behavioral Research. *Deciding to Forego Life-Sustaining Treatment.* Washington, DC: US Government Printing Office; 1983.

XX. PERSISTENT VEGETATIVE STATE (PVS)

DEFINITION
Total loss of cerebral cortical function with a functioning brain stem.

CHARACTERISTICS OF PVS
1. Sleep-like coma for a few days to a few weeks. Then the eyes open, and sleep-wake cycles begin.
2. "Eyes-open unconsciousness." Eyes move in random fashion but do not focus or follow. Patient is "awake but unaware." (In cases other than PVS, when recovery does occur, true tracking of objects by the eyes is often the first sign of recovery. This must be differentiated from a brief turning of the eyes of the PVS patient toward the source of sound, which is a primitive reflex.)
3. Unintelligible grunts, screams; grimacing and chewing without purpose. Swallowing is uncoordinated, so the patient must be tube fed.
4. Many reflexes are present including corneal, cough, gag, and startle.
5. The presence of gross involuntary, reflexive movement without purpose.

PROGNOSIS AND DIAGNOSIS
After 3 months, the prognosis for recovery is virtually nil. It may be possible to establish lack of recovery of independent function after 1 month in patients whose PVS is caused by cerebral hypoxia.

The diagnosis is clinical; no definitive laboratory test is available. Neurological consultation should be obtained for confirmation. PVS is not recognized in law as "death."

NURSING CARE AND MANAGEMENT
1. Good communication is required to help the family to understand that the patient, by definition, cannot be suffering. Sensations such as pain, hunger, thirst, and suffering—just like joy and awareness—are cortically mediated and are absent in PVS.
2. Usually the patient is not ventilator dependent, so the decision may be about whether to withdraw fluid and nutrition. This deter-

mination is easier to make if the patient has an advance directive or a reliable, informed surrogate decision maker.

FURTHER READING

Prognosis of PVS

One study reported that, following cerebral hypoxia-ischemia (the most common cause of PVS), no patient who remained vegetative for more than 1 month ever regained consciousness (*JAMA*. 1985;253:1420-1426). Some states require a period of 3 months in PVS for a definitive diagnosis. The prognosis depends on the circumstances; in young adults and in cases of subarachnoid hemorrhage, it may take longer to predict the inability to recover independent function.

The general rules to establish a "hopeless" prognosis are:
1.   3 months after hypoxic episode in child or young adult
2.   12 months after head injury in a child
3.   6 months after head injury in an adult

After these intervals, recovery is extremely unlikely. Those few who recover remain nursing-home patients with severe neurologic deficit, including the "locked-in" syndrome.

Prognosis in the Coma Phase Following Hypoxic-Ischemic Brain Injury

Patients who will not regain independent function have the following characteristics:
1.   No pupillary light reflexes at time of initial exam
2.   Lack of corneal reflexes after the first day
3.   Persistence of coma at 7 days
4.   The absence of oculocephalic reflexes or the absence of purposeful motor response to pain portend a poor prognosis.

Laboratory Studies in PVS

Although there are no definitive studies, positron emission tomography (PET) scans of PVS patients have shown cortical glucose consumption to be at the same low level as that of patients in deep anesthesia. Serial computed tomography (CT) scans show significant and progressive atrophy but no specific changes. Autopsy studies routinely show bilateral hemispheric damage to a degree that is incompatible with consciousness.

REFERENCES

American Medical Association, Council on Scientific Affairs and Council on Ethical and Judicial Affairs. Persistent vegetative state and the decision to withdraw or withhold life support. *JAMA*. 1990;263:426-430.

Cranford RE. The persistent vegetative state: the medical reality (getting the facts straight). *Hastings Cent Rep*. 1988;18:27-32.

Crispi F, Crisci C. Patients in persistent vegetative state . . . and what of their relatives? *Nurs*

Ethics. 2000;7:533-535.

Levy DE, et al. Predicting outcome from hypoxic ischemic coma. *JAMA.* 1985;253:1420-1426.

Perkins EM. Speak up! Death can be a caring choice. *RN.* 1998;61(2):72.

Sadala MLA, Mendes HWB. Caring for organ donors: the intensive care unit nurses' view. *Qualitative Health Res.* 2000;10:788-805.

Suk H. The ethical dilemma of patients in a vegetative state. *Int Nurs Rev.* 1998;45(5):142.

Waldon AF, Hubbell CL, Taylor TC. Nurses shouldn't stand in the way of patients' wishes: "Killing, not caring." *RN.* 1997;60(8):9.

XXI. AUTOPSY

NEED FOR AUTOPSIES

Nurses and physicians sometimes think autopsies are no longer necessary in this era of computed tomography and magnetic resonance imaging. Autopsies are still needed, however, for medical, legal, epidemiological, and familial reasons.

INDICATIONS FOR AUTOPSY

1. Comply with medical examiner's requirements
2. Clarify puzzling cases
3. Delineate suspected or unsuspected medical conditions
4. Provide useful information to the family
5. Reassure survivors with negative findings
6. Collect statistical data
7. Define environmental and occupational hazards
8. Provide legal and forensic information
9. Enhance clinical, pathological, and medical education

MEDICAL EXAMINER CASES

These are cases that must, by law, be reported to the medical examiner:

1. Unexplained or unusual circumstances surrounding death
2. All homicides
3. All suicides
4. All deaths following abortion
5. All deaths due to poisoning (homicidal, suicidal, or accidental)
6. All deaths following accidents, regardless of whether the injury was the primary cause of death. (For example, a patient hospitalized for treatment of fractures sustained in an automobile accident who dies in the hospital of a myocardial infarction still needs to be reported.)
7. When no physician is in attendance
8. When the attending physician refuses to sign the death certificate

If there is doubt about the need to report, it is best to call the medical examiner's office.

NOTIFYING AND COUNSELING THE FAMILY

Immediately after pronouncing death:

1. Notify the attending physician and determine if he or she wishes to inform the family.
2. If the task is delegated to you, speak in person to the family, if possible.
3. Avoid giving this information over the phone—do it only if necessary.
4. Identify yourself as the nurse caring for the family's loved one.
5. Inform them gently that the patient has died and avoid euphemisms such as "passed away" and "expired."
6. Express sympathy. Physical contact such as a hand on the shoulder may be appropriate.
7. If appropriate to the situation, you may wish to involve the hospital chaplain, social worker, or other staff members that the family may have become close to and feel comfortable talking with.
8. Usually the physician sensitively discusses the question of autopsy, giving the reasons for its importance in this case (such as uncertainty of diagnosis, the family's need to know, scientific advancement). Nurses often relay the family members' wishes to the physicians in matters of request for autopsy.
9. The family can be assured that an open-casket funeral service is not precluded by the procedure.
10. Check with your institution as to whether the autopsy can be done without charge to the family members.

OBTAINING CONSENT FOR AN AUTOPSY

Phone consent is not valid. Consent for the autopsy must be obtained in writing, by telegram, or by fax. Related costs may or may not be provided by the hospital or insurance provider. Advise the family to review payment options at the institution. Consent should be obtained from the next of kin in the following order:

1. Surviving spouse. If none, then
2. Adult children. If none, then
3. Parents. If none, then
4. Brothers and sisters. If none, then
5. Any relative (or friend) who assumes custody of the body
6. If none of the above can be found 48 hours after death, hospital administration can give consent.

If the case is reported to the medical examiner and accepted for autopsy, family consent is not necessary; the family has no option for refusal. Furthermore, a consent signed by any agent listed above does not preclude an autopsy by the medical examiner.

AFTER THE DEATH

1. You may want to attend the funeral (if your relationship to the patient makes this appropriate).
2. If you were close with the patient, it is appropriate to send a card or a brief letter.
3. Many institutions are now offering a bereavement service to families and caregivers alike. Encourage the use of such a service if one is available.
4. If an autopsy was performed, the family members can be informed that pathologists are also available for consultation and that written autopsy reports are usually available within four to six weeks of the procedure. A family can also obtain a copy of the report by contacting the physician or institution.

REFERENCES

Gonzalez C. The influence of culture in the authorization of an autopsy. *J Clin Ethics*. 1993;4:192-194.

Orlowski JP, Vinicky JK. Conflicting cultural attitudes about autopsies. *J Clin Ethics*. 1993;4:195-197.

Perkins HS, Supik JD, Hazuda HP. Autopsy decisions: the possibility of conflicting cultural attitudes. *J Clin Ethics*. 1993;4:145-154.

Rosenbaum G, et al. Autopsy consent practice at US teaching hospitals: results of a national survey. *Arch Intern Med*. 2000;160: 374-380.

XXII. CULTURAL COMPETENCE

IMPLICATIONS FOR NURSES

In order to provide care that is culturally relevant to a diverse patient population, nurses must be aware of and sensitive to the values, beliefs, and health practices of different cultures. According to Leninger, culturally competent care is "a complex integration of knowledge, attitudes and skill that enhances cross cultural communication and appropriate and effective interaction with others." In many instances, nurses provide care across cultures, so it is an ethical imperative for nurses to develop the skill of culturally competent caring.

To care for patients of other cultures effectively, the nurse must be a conscientious observer and a perceptive listener and assessor. Acquiring information about the patient's culture and gaining further personal insight helps the nurse to provide culturally competent care. Some cultures vary in orientation to time. This behavior may be noted in scheduling medical appointments.

Variations in communication patterns may be evidenced in different cultures. Patterns may vary in:
1. Tone or volume
2. Direct/indirect communication
3. Direction of eye gaze (may be perceived as intimidating or disrespectful)
4. Physical distance between speakers
5. Gestures made while speaking

STRATEGIES FOR SELF-DEVELOPMENT
1. Learn from cultural encounters
2. Record your observations
3. Listen and learn from others
4. Identify and document patterns
5. Validate your observations and learning
6. Attend cultural events
7. Read articles on cultural competence
8. Contact local colleges for speakers or colleagues to provide cultural training

9. Access the Internet

The need for culturally competent care can be addressed through education and self-reflection. Self-reflection allows the nurse to examine his or her own reasons for any underlying assumptions that may be evidenced in the nurse-patient relationship. Nursing administrators, managers, and educators are discovering the critical need to have knowledge and skills related to multicultural care to serve patients.

Nurses, as individuals, bring to their practice assumptions from their own culture as well as assumptions about the cultures of others. Cultural diversity is the current standard, and nursing staff development programs that are sensitive to this fact produce employees with advantages over those from settings that do not prepare staff for practice in a constantly changing world.

REFERENCES

Doswell WM, Erlen JA. Multicultural issues and ethical concerns in the delivery of nursing care interventions. *Nurs Clin North Am*. 1998;2:353-361.

Hui E. Chinese health care ethics. In: Coward H, Ratanakul P, eds. *A Cross-Cultural Dialogue on Health Care Ethics*. Waterloo, Ont: Wilfrid Laurier University Press;1999.

Leninger M. *Cultural Care: Diversity and Universality: A Theory of Nursing*. New York: National League for Nursing Press; 1996.

Leninger M. Transcultural nursing education: a worldwide imperative. *Nursing & Health Care*. 1994;5:254-257.

Mahon P. Transcultural nursing: a source guide. *J Nurs Staff Dev*. 1997;13(4):218-222.

XXIII. RESEARCH

ETHICAL ISSUES

Clinical research is performed in a variety of healthcare settings including hospitals, clinics, and labs. Nurses who work with any stage of research involving human subjects must be aware of the following ethical guidelines:

1. The design of the research study must be ethical—that is, the risks cannot outweigh the potential benefits to society or to the individual.
2. The selection of participants for the study must reflect an unbiased, nonjudgmental approach on the part of the researcher. For example, participants should not consist of all males or all females unless the protocol is studying a related phenomenon.
3. All research participants must give consent. They must have decision-making capacity, give their consent freely, and be informed appropriately.
4. The consent form should be written at approximately an eighth-grade reading level.
5. The consent form should be translated into other languages as appropriate.
6. Confidentiality should be emphasized throughout the research protocol and the consent process.
7. The researcher(s) must obtain approval from the institutional review board (IRB) for protocols involving human participants. The purpose of IRB review is to ensure protection of human subjects in research.
8. Ideally, conflicts of interest should not be present. If they are present, they must be disclosed to the participants.
9. Stipends for participation should not be so large that they could be construed as "coercive" or as undue influence in recruitment of participants.
10. Participants must be free to quit the study protocol at any time during the research process.

NURSES' ROLE IN CLINICAL RESEARCH

The humans that are subjects in clinical trials used to be called "subjects." Because that term may seem cold and dehumanizing, we now refer to humans in research as "participants."

Nurses may function as primary investigators, or they may be asked to assist in the facilitation of clinical research via data collection (such as compiling patient records or talking with patients). It is important that researchers inform nurses about the study protocol and provide instructions about nurses' expected role before the study is initiated. For example, if nurses are expected to collect tissue specimens from patients, they must know how to gather, store, and transport the specimen so as not to contaminate it or make an error. Additionally, nurses must be able to check that patients have consented for participation in the research study and to assess whether patients have questions or require further explanation. Nurses need to know who the primary investigators are and how to contact them.

At times, nurses may be involved in studies using a placebo. Again, it is imperative for the researchers to discuss their protocol in advance with nursing staff so that concerns may be addressed before data collection begins.

REFERENCES

Davis AJ. Informed consent process in research protocols: dilemmas for clinical nurses." *Western J Nurs Res.* 1989;11(4):448-457.

Engelking C. Facilitating clinical trials: the expanding role of the nurse. *Cancer* 1991;67(6):1793-1797.

Glenister D. Focus. Nursing research ethics: some problems and recommended changes. *Nursing Times Research* 1996;1(3):184-90.

Kelly PJ, Cordell J. Recruitment of women into research studies: a nursing perspective. *Clin Nurse Spec.* 1996;10(1):25-28.

Kjervik DK, Penticuff J. The future of nursing research in ethics and law. *J Prof Nurs.* 1992;8(3):141.

Lowes L. Paediatric nursing and research ethics: is there a conflict? *J Clin Nurs.* 1996;5(2):91-7.

Namei S, et al. The ethics of role conflict in research. *J Neuroscie Nurs.* 1993;25:326-330.

Sadler GR, et al. Nurses' unique roles in randomized clinical trials. *J Prof Nurs.* 1999;15(2):106-115.

Wolfe S. Legally speaking. Clinical trials: how informed should consent be? *RN.* 2000;63(6):77-82.

XXIV. ETHICS CONSULTATION

ETHICS COMMITTEES

Institutional ethics committees (ECs) have a variety of configurations. Many are standing committees of the medical staff, which report to the medical executive committee or governing staff of the hospital. Most meet monthly, or more frequently as occasion demands. Some institutions that do not have large ECs contract with ethicists, or other trained individuals, outside of the organization. Typically ECs have three tasks:

1. Education—of committee members, staff, and community
2. Policy formulation—the EC is not a policy-making body, but will suggest policy on request of the medical staff or hospital administration
3. Case consultation—on request

REASONS FOR CASE CONSULTATION

An ethics consultation might be considered for some of the following reasons:

1. For clarification of issues regarding decision-making capacity, informed consent, or advance directives
2. To provide recommendations for cases involving do-not-resuscitate orders or withdrawal of treatment
3. To help in resolution of ethical conflict—between family and caregivers, patient and caregivers, patient and family, or among staff members

THE NURSE AS BIOETHICS CONSULTANT

Nurse bioethics consultants should have substantial patient care and clinical experience, instruction in case law, and knowledge of humanistic behavior. The additional education and training necessary to act as a bioethics consultant may be obtained through selected master's or doctoral programs. In some areas of the United States, certificate programs that focus on bioethics in healthcare are offered.

An important aspect of the consultant's training is the clinical experience of consultation at the bedside or at the committee level. Interpersonal skills, such as communication and interviewing, are essential for the proficient consultant. In addition, the bioethics consultant must be knowledgeable in philosophy, healthcare law, public policy, and medical terminology and treatments in order to demonstrate competence in this advanced practice role.

The bioethics consultant is considered a collegial member of the healthcare team, and he or she often functions as a member of an institutional EC as well. The purpose of the EC is to provide education, act as a resource, and identify referral needs in relation to nursing practice issues and or ethical dilemmas as they affect patients care. The importance of a nurse ethicist on the EC cannot be overstated.

Many hospitals have had institutional or medical ECs since the early 1980s. This type of EC focuses mainly on policy development and review, administrative functions, and case consultation. These hospital-level committees usually consist of physicians, administrators, social workers, lawyers, laypersons, bioethicists, and nurses. The importance of a nurse ethicist on such an EC cannot be overstated.

Institutional ECs are not always the most conducive means of addressing questions or concerns in nursing ethics. Nursing ECs, comprised primarily of nurses, may be the most appropriate strategy for nurses to examine the ethical dilemmas that arise in their daily patient care activities. Participation on nursing ECs promotes nurses' moral reasoning, enhances their ethical decision-making and patient-advocacy skills, and increases their professional satisfaction. Such a committee also provides education for other nurses in philosophical ethics, ethical principles, decision-making skills, and group interaction processes. The nurse ethicist on such a committee can assist nurses in their role as patient advocates.

The nurse ethicist also serves to advance nursing ethics research and may provide direction to the nursing EC to guide future research. The nurse ethicist can make recommendations and provide insight into the feasibility of specific nursing ethics research projects. Nurses are an integral part of any patient's hospital care and are often the first to note ethical concerns related to a patient's care. The nurse who has gained experience on a nursing EC will be better prepared to assist patients during this critical time.

The nurse ethicist's clinical skills include the ability to:

1. Identify and analyze moral problems in a specific patient's case
2. Use reasonable clinical judgment in solving ethical conflicts
3. Communicate effectively with healthcare professionals, patients, and families
4. Negotiate and facilitate negotiations
5. Teach other healthcare professionals how to identify, analyze, and resolve similar problems in similar cases

FURTHER READING

Case Consultation Method
(This is the approach used by the authors' institutional EC.)

1. **Response to Consultation Request**

   The consultant(s) or the EC member(s) who initially responds to the request for consultation should consider the following:

   - Who requested the consult? If it was not the attending physician, does he or she agree?
   - What is the ethical problem? Is the problem ethical—or does it involve legal, social, or psychological issues; staff conflict; or miscommunication? Is it a problem that needs referral to another service?
   - What specifically is being requested of the EC? Clarification of the problem? Mediation? Recommendations?

2. **Evaluation by the Responding Consultant**

   - See the patient. If patient has decision-making capacity, notify him or her of the nature of the visit and ask permission. If the patient does not have decision-making capacity, seek the permission of the guardian or healthcare agent.
   - Interview the patient.
   - Interview nursing personnel, other personnel, and family members.
   - Discuss the problem with the attending physician and other consultants.
   - Review the chart.

3. **Decision about Emergency Meeting of Full EC**

   - If the problem is uncomplicated, common, and the reaction of the EC can be anticipated, the consultant may resolve it.
   - If the problem is unusual, complicated, problematic, or delicate, a full EC meeting is called.

4. **Assessment of the Ethical Problem(s)**

   (By either the initial consultant(s) or the entire EC)

- **Medical Facts**
  - Decision-making capacity of the patient
  - Current medical status, diagnosis, and prognosis
  - Recommended treatment and reasonable alternative treatments
  - Effect of no treatment
  - Assessment of the patient's life expectancy
  - Views of caregivers
- **Patient's Preference**
  - Has the patient been informed and given time to reflect on options?
  - What are the patient's personal/social factors? What is his or her value system?
  - What is the patient's personal assessment of quality of life?
  - What are the patient's current expressed choices?
  - Are there any advance directives?
- **External Factors**
  - Family:
    - How well do they know and represent the patient?
    - Do they understand the situation? Are they in agreement?
    - Is there any conflict of interest?
  - If there is no advance directive, who is the decision maker?
  - Religion—Are religious values involved?
  - Cultural—Are cultural issues involved?
  - Expense—Is it a factor in the patient's decisions?
  - Legal issues—Are there applicable hospital policies or state statutes?

5. **Problem Resolution**
   - Make sure the information is complete.
   - Delineate the ethical problem clearly.
   - Clarify the options.
     - Did we ensure as much patient autonomy as possible?
     - Are our recommendations consistent with the patient's preferences or best interest?
     - Are our recommendations consistent with ethical principles?

6. **Reporting**
   - Recommendations are made as recommendations. It is up to the attending physician to take or reject them, as is true of all consultations.
   - Report of the consultation will be placed on the chart, if requested.
   - Full report of the consultation will be detailed in the minutes of the EC.
   - Full minutes as required by medical staff bylaws will go to the medical staff executive committee.

7. **Follow Up**
   In many situations, the consultant(s) will need to follow the patient in order to be available for further consultation. In this way, the consultant can check on the patient's status and make progress reports to the EC for educational purposes.

REFERENCES

Fletcher JC, Siegler M. What are the goals of ethics consultation? A consensus statement. *J Clin Ethics*. 1996;7:122-126.

Jonsen AR. Case analysis in clinical ethics. *J Clin Ethics*. 1990;1:63-65.

La Puma J, Schiedermayer D. *Ethics Consultation: A Practical Guide*. Boston: Jones and Bartlett; 1994.

Schroeter, K. Perioperative involvement on nursing ethics committees. *AORN J*.1996;64(4)588-596.

Schroeter, K. Expanded practice: the nurse as bioethics consultant. *Semin Perioperative Nurs*. 2000;9:65-70.

Singer PA, Pellegrino ED, Siegler M. Ethics committees and consultants. *J Clin Ethics*. 1989;1:263-267.

Walker MU. Keeping moral spaces open: new images of ethics consulting. *Hastings Cent Rep*. 1993;23:33-40.

XXV. ETHICS AND MANAGED CARE

In today's healthcare system, all care is managed to some extent or another. Many nurses have some contact with or work for some type of managed-care organization (MCO) either full time or at least part time. Managed care and capitation have introduced new stressors into the practice of nursing and into the relationship between healthcare providers and their patients.

NEW PRESSURES ON NURSES

1. **Divided Loyalties**

   The traditional role of the nurse as patient advocate must be balanced against the need to save money for the organization. The major question is whether the nurse can function in this role without compromising patient care and patient welfare. For example, MCOs often require nurses to carry too high of a patient load or working consecutive shifts without adequate relief.

2. **Limited Tests and Treatments**

   The American Medical Association Council on Ethical and Judicial Affairs has issued the following statement: "As part of the process of giving patients informed consent to treatment, physicians should disclose all available treatment alternatives, regardless of cost, including those potentially beneficial treatments that are not offered under the terms of the plan" (*JAMA*. 1995;273:330-335).

   Patients need to be aware that limitations of interventions (testing and treatment) should be dictated by their disease process rather than by the rules of the MCO. If a second-best but less expensive antibiotic is prescribed because of the provider restrictions of the MCO formulary, patients need to know this (and either accept it, challenge it with their provider, or seek other insurance coverage options).

3. **Limited Choice of Physician/Specialist/Institution Referral**

   One real benefit of managed-care systems may be the establishment of a primary care physician who provides continuity of care, serves as a ready source of contact, and makes appropriate referrals for care beyond his or her expertise.

Problems can occur if the primary care provider does not have on-going responsibility (for example, if the patient sees a different provider at each visit), if the primary care provider is pushed beyond his or her level of expertise in order to avoid expensive referral, or if the primary provider is allowed to refer only to MCO physicians when a far superior specialist for a particular problem is in the community but not associated with the MCO. Additionally, patients may be forced to travel great distances to see their primary provider or specialist and/or to obtain treatment at a participating facility.

PROBLEMS INHERENT IN THE MCO

1. **Administrative Costs and Profit Taking**

   Most MCOs are for-profit entities with stockholders who must be paid. In such MCOs, about 74% of revenues are returned to healthcare; the remainder goes to investor profits, administrative costs, and executive salaries.

2. **Patient and Provider "Churning"**

   Patients are moved from doctor to doctor and system to system. Sometimes a patient may be forced to change healthcare systems several times even while employed at the same job. Similarly, doctors and healthcare organizations join and leave MCOs abruptly. All of these changes disrupt the patient-doctor-nurse-clinic-hospital relationship.

3. **Confidentiality**

   Preservation of confidentiality of patient information is increasingly difficult with computerized records being shared within and between organizations.

4. **Provision of Care to Indigent Patients or Support for Medical Education or Research**

   MCOs, with a few notable exceptions, lack an educational mission and avoid involvement with teaching hospitals and institutions that provide care for indigent patients.

PRACTICE GUIDELINES

Guidelines must be flexible, scientifically legitimate, and widely accepted by professional medical organizations. Guidelines should remain *guidelines* and not become *requirements*. They should allow for some variability to accommodate unique clinical circumstances, because not all patients present with classical textbook symptoms or fit neatly into protocols.

Practice guidelines can be very helpful in avoiding marginally useful or unhelpful interventions and tests. However, they can also become restrictive, and have been referred to as "cookbook medicine." Guidelines must be reassessed and revised periodically by physicians to avoid becoming outdated recipes.

RATIONING

Macro-allocation refers to the way resources are allocated to groups of people—to the entire MCO or to society as a whole. The lives involved are faceless and statistical. *Micro-allocation* refers to the situation in which people deal with one another on a one-to-one basis; the lives are identified lives. Rationing at this level is "bedside rationing." According to the American Medical Association, allocation judgments about costs and services that approach a "rationing" decision (such as the denial of a procedure that benefits a patient) are not part of the physician's traditional role and, indeed, conflict with it (*JAMA*. 1995;273:330-335).

Similarly, nurses should not be involved in the process of micro-allocation. At the bedside or in the clinic, the only responsibility of the ethical nurse is to act as an advocate for the patient. If distribution of healthcare resources is to be fair and just, rationing decisions must be made by society so that any limits imposed on patients are shared by all healthcare providers and patients in the same clinical setting.

On the other hand, nurses and physicians should be involved in the process of macro-allocation. It is their duty as good citizens—a duty made even more important by the special knowledge that they bring to the deliberations. Nurses abrogate their public responsibility if they allow bureaucrats or nonprofessional individuals to make policy decisions without their emphatic input.

CAN THE ETHICAL NURSE-PATIENT RELATIONSHIP ENDURE IN THE MANAGED-CARE MILIEU?

The answer can be yes, but only under certain conditions.

1. The MCO should allow full informed consent. Patients should be informed of all appropriate interventions for their medical problems, including those not offered by the MCO contract.

2. Healthcare providers' salaries should not be individually predicated only on saving the MCO money, but should also be based on the quality of care rendered. If there is a small incentive bonus, it should be truly small and patients should be aware of it.

3. If there are MCO practice guidelines, there should be allowance for deviation under unusual circumstances and frequent physician-directed revision to reflect new scientific evidence.

4. In short, the participating nurses must be allowed as much latitude as possible in exercising their primary responsibility— fulfilling the trust of their patients that their acts of caring are motivated only by concern for patients' welfare.

REFERENCES

American Medical Association, Council on Ethical and Judicial Affairs. Ethical issues in managed care. *JAMA*. 1995;273:330-335.

Crawshaw R, et al. The patient-physician covenant. *JAMA*. 1995;273:1553.

Daniels N. *Just Health Care*. New York: Cambridge University Press; 1985.

Ginsberg E, Ostow M. Managed care: a look back and a look ahead. *N Engl J Med*. 1997;336:1018-1020.

Gostin LO, et al. Privacy and security of personal information in a new health care system. *JAMA*. 1993;270:2487-2493.

Jecker NS, Jonsen AR. Healthcare as a commons. *Cambridge Q Healthcare Ethics*. 1995;4:207-216.

Kassirer JP. Is managed care here to stay? *N Engl J Med*. 1997;336:1013-1014.

Kerr EA, et al. Primary care physicians' satisfaction with quality of care in California capitated medical groups. *JAMA*. 1997;278:308-312.

Swartz K, Brennan TA. Integrated health care, capitated payment and quality: the role of regulation. *Ann Intern Med*. 1996;124:442-448.

Weingarten S. Practice guidelines and predication rules should be subject to careful clinical testing. *JAMA*. 1997;277:1977-1978.

XXVI. BIOETHICS:
THEORIES AND PRINCIPLES

THEORIES

Ethics, as a branch of philosophy, has been studied since ancient times. Bioethics, on the other hand, is a relatively new field originating in the 1970s and gaining momentum until the present day. When nurses and other healthcare providers are involved in ethical decision making, not everyone analyzes the issues from a similar view. There are many theories that are used to help us evaluate ethical issues. Ethical theories consider the motive or intent of the practitioner/agent (the choice to do something or the will), the means used by the agent to accomplish the act (the way something is done), and the consequences of the act (the end or the results from the action). A few of the more commonly used theories are listed here:

1. **Utilitarianism**

    The basic premise of utilitarianism is that ethical conflicts may be resolved by considering the number of individuals affected by the decision (the greatest good for the greatest number). An action or means of practice is right if it focuses on maximizing the good consequences and minimizing the bad consequences as a whole.

2. **Deontology**

    This theory is based on the concept of duty or binding obligation. The means of an action are intrinsically or inherently right or wrong. Nurses are bound by their professional duty to always do right by their patients. In essence, nurses do what is good for their patients because it is the nurse's duty to care for patients properly.

3. **Virtue**

    Virtue theory evolved from the philosophy of Aristotle. The intent of the agent (person taking the ethical stand or action) is what determines whether or not the act is good or moral. If the intent is to do good, then the act is considered ethical—even if the outcome is bad.

4. **Egoist**

Objectivism, a philosophy developed in the latter half of the 20th century, puts forth an ethical theory or system of rational self-interest. It does not treat ethics as an isolated field, but builds on two prerequisite branches of philosophy: metaphysics (our world around us) and epistemology (how we know what we know). Although this growing philosophical movement carries with it some controversy, such as selfishness as a virtue, it deserves investigation.

PRINCIPLES

The American Nurses Association code for nurses uses the four principles of bioethics as identified by Beauchamp and Childress (autonomy, beneficence, nonmaleficence, and justice). The principles of veracity and fidelity are also used in resolving ethical issues in healthcare. In many cases, healthcare providers must choose between conflicting principles.

1. **Autonomy**

Autonomy is the self-determination of an individual, encompassing respect for persons. Healthcare providers are obligated to respect the right of patients to make voluntary, uncoerced decisions about life situations.

2. **Beneficence**

Beneficence is the principle of doing good. Healthcare providers are obligated to do good for their patients, to benefit or to act in the best interest of patients.

3. **Nonmaleficence**

Healthcare providers are obligated to do no harm.

4. **Justice**

Patients have the right to be treated fairly and to receive equal care.

5. **Veracity**

Veracity is the principle of truth-telling. Healthcare providers are expected to be truthful about all aspects of the patient's care.

6.   **Fidelity**

Healthcare providers are obligated to keep their promises to the patient and maintain the confidentiality of patient information.

APPLICATION TO PRACTICE

A variety of approaches can be used to deal with ethical dilemmas.

1.   **Principlism**

The *principlist* approach uses the afore-mentioned principles to represent and codify certain values and understandings of ethics. Depending on the situation, one or more principles may take precedence over the others. The interaction between the principles will generate a resolution to the conflict, and the interaction will vary depending on the dynamics of the ethical situation encountered.

2.   **Casuistry**

The approach known as *casuistry* works on the premise that we can reflect upon the practices and situations of routine daily living and social institutions in which the right actions are clear or paradigmatic. Concepts or principles are the byproduct of the analysis of given cases. Casuistry emphasizes practical problem-solving by means of subtle interpretations of individual cases based on paradigm cases. The cases used are real, and it is important that they are long, richly detailed, and comprehensive in order to promote the best understanding. Additionally, the cases should reflect the perspectives of all the involved participants. Ethical principles are applied in casuistry, but are discovered in the cases themselves and are identified gradually after reflecting upon particular cases.

The strength of the ethical perspective is its prescriptive nature. It promotes an action guide for nurses to follow in the realm of patient care. Because ethics is a branch of philosophy, multiple approaches can be taken when applying ethics to real-life situations. Thus, each nurse may experience a situation differently, in terms of identifying the ethical issues, feelings, behaviors, actions, analysis, and resolution of the situation.

REFERENCES

American Hospital Association. A patient's bill of rights. In: Reich WT, ed. *Encyclopedia of Bioethics.* New York: McMillan; 1978:4:1782-1783.

Beauchamp TL, Childress JF, *Principles of Biomedical Ethics.* 4th ed. New York: Oxford University Press; 1994:436-437.

Edwards SD, What are the limits to the obligations of the nurse? *J Med Ethics.* 1996;2:90-94.

Fry ST, *Ethics in Nursing Practice: A Guide to Ethical Decision Making.* Geneva: International Council of Nurses; 1994.

McDaniel C. Enhancing nurses' ethical practice. *Nurs Clin North Am.* 1998;2:299-311.

Peikoff L. *Objectivism: The Philosophy of Ayn Rand.* New York: Dutton; 1991.

Prins MM. Patient advocacy: The role of nursing leadership. *Nursg Manage.* 1992;7:78-80.

Willard C. The nurse's role as patient advocate: obligation or imposition? *J Adv Nurs.* 1996;24:60-66.

XXVII. THE FUTURE OF ETHICS IN NURSING: IMPLICATIONS FOR NURSE MANAGERS

It is important for nurses to be proactive when it comes to ethics. Nurse managers can make staff members aware of ethical issues in a variety of ways.

1. The manager can provide clarification in an open-forum discussion or at staff meetings. Discussing, identifying, and addressing the ethical issues will promote a more cohesive work group. Nurses will feel more comfortable handling the issues because they understand the protocols to be taken in the clinical setting.

2. A departmental focus group can be developed to allow staff to identify the most important issues. The manager, or designee, can serve as a facilitator in these discussions to bring issues out into the open and encourage staff to brainstorm on the most effective means of dealing with the issues.

3. Nurse managers can enhance their understanding of bioethics issues by reading articles and making contacts within professional organizations.

4. Some staff members may have a more difficult time than others dealing with ethical issues. It may be necessary for the manager to counsel these people individually. Sometimes, it is a matter of helping them deal with conflict. It is important that the manager provide support to the staff. Nursing staff members need to know that if they encounter a situation involving ethical conflict, their manager will support them.

5. To enhance nurses' understanding of issues in medical ethics, the nurse manager can encourage staff to become involved as members of the nursing or medical ethics committee. Membership on such a committee can help nurses obtain the knowledge and skills necessary to assist patients and peers in ethical decision making. Participation improves nurses' moral reasoning, enhances their ethical decision-making and patient-advocacy skills, and increases their professional satisfaction.

6. Nurse managers can encourage their organization to review

and develop policies and procedures to address the types of ethical situations occurring in practice.

7. Because nurse administrators are in positions of influence in their organizations and communities, they have the responsibility to assume leadership in increasing nursing's voice and visibility in changing the system and influencing health policy.

IMPLICATIONS FOR CLINICIANS

1. Each nurse must be familiar with the ethical issues. To learn more about the issues, nurses can discuss them with peers or with ethics committee members.

2. It is beneficial for nurses to have a file on ethics available in the department for review.

3. Departments can offer inservice training on ethical issues by using members of the hospital's nursing ethics or medical ethics committees.

4. The social services department can provide assistance, especially in the area of advance directives.

5. Values clarification can help nurses identify and understand their moral beliefs and attitudes. When the nursing environment is too fraught with conflict, some nurses choose to work in another area of healthcare or leave the profession entirely.

6. It is imperative for nurses to develop and adhere to protocols for dealing with ethical dilemmas in their specific practice environment.

CONCLUSION

As healthcare shifts toward a more cost-oriented focus, it is imperative for nurses and other healthcare providers to understand the concepts and issues that affect patient care. Nurses must develop an understanding of ethics terminology and considerations that will enable them to manage such situations in the future.

Nursing combines high-tech care with high-touch care into a highly specialized profession. Nurses in any specialty area cannot deny their responsibility and accountability to their patients. It is no longer enough simply to "do no harm." Today's nurses must ensure that safe, competent, legal, and ethical care is provided to all patients. Ethical practice is a critical aspect of nursing care, and the development of ethical competency should be paramount for present and future nursing practice.

REFERENCES

American Nurses Association. *Code of Ethics for Nurses with Interpretive Statements.* Kansas City, Mo: ANA; 2001.

Kobs A. Questions & answers from the JCAHO. Ethics and patients' rights. *Nurs Manage.* July 1997;7:20.

Schroeter K. Ethics for surgical services managers: now and in the future. *Surg Serv Manage.* 1997;3(8):32-35.